D0114220

EQUAL PARTNERS

EQUAL PARTNERS

A Physician's Call for a New Spirit of Medicine

Jody Heymann, M.D.

LITTLE, BROWN AND COMPANY

BOSTON   NEW YORK   TORONTO   LONDON

The author is grateful for permission to include the following previously copyrighted
material:

Excerpt from "Dreams" from *The Dream Keeper and Other Poems* by Langston Hughes.
Copyright 1932 by Alfred A. Knopf Inc. and © renewed 1960 by Langston Hughes.
Reprinted by permission of the publisher.

Library of Congress Cataloging-in-Publication Data

Heymann, Jody.
    Equal partners : a physician's call for a new spirit of medicine /
Jody Heymann. — 1st ed.
        p.   cm.
    Includes bibliographical references.
    ISBN 0-316-35993-9
    1. Heymann, Jody — Health.   2. Brain — Hemorrhage — Patients —
United States — Biography.   3. Hemangioma — Patients — United States —
Biography.   4. Physicians — United States — Biography.   5. Physician
and patient — United States.   6. Medical care — United States.
I. Title.
    [DNLM: 1. Physician-Patient Relations — personal narratives.
2. Informed Consent — personal narratives.   WZ 100 H6175 1994]
RC394.H37H49   1994
610.69'6 — dc20
[B]
DNLM/DLC
for Library of Congress   94-31936

10   9   8   7   6   5   4   3   2   1

MV-NY

Published simultaneously in Canada by Little, Brown & Company (Canada) Limited

Printed in the United States of America

To T., B., and J.

Whose love got me through
and made it all worthwhile

Contents

Acknowledgments

LIKE MANY PIECES of work, this book is the outgrowth of the efforts of many people, although the responsibility for its contents rests on my shoulders.

I am forever grateful to the family, friends, and physicians who got me through the medical experiences I had as a patient. Without them, there would have been no starting point from which to return to work. The book tells about a fraction of their kindnesses and support, the patient and professional care they provided. Their names — with the exception of my immediate family — have been changed in the book to allow them to keep their privacy.

When I fell, my family helped me believe I could get back on my feet. With love, humor, and faith, my husband, Tim, got me through the worst hours of pain and the longest months of doubt. My brother, Steve, had long taught me by the example that is his life not to let physical challenges get in the way of dreams or commitment. My parents had given us their enduring love and encouragement that we should each try to do something meaningful with our lives. My uncle helped teach me how little the risks of seizures ultimately had to limit my life.

When I was ready to return to work, I was fortunate to have supervisors filled with patience and courage instead of discrimination. No physician makes it through internship without a great deal of support from colleagues — physicians, nurses, and social workers. The work I was able to do at Children's Hospital, and since, owes a great debt to them.

I am equally deeply indebted to the many patients and their families who shared their lives with me. Their profound courage, endurance, kindness, and humanity will always stay with me. Like those of physicians, patients' names have been changed as have potentially identifying characteristics to allow them to keep their privacy.

When I began writing this book, Linda Bauer and Hannah Mahoney read early drafts. They gave invaluable time, encouragement, and greatly needed advice. Without them, this book would not have come to be.

Charlotte Sheedy made a dream into a possibility. As a literary agent she provided critical advice and ever available support. Throughout this project, I repeatedly counted my blessings — that Charlotte and my editor, Jim Silberman, were working with me. The extent to which this book is a "first book" is because of me; the extent to which it is a good book is because of Jim. To make the book more readable, he advised me to let the story raise the policy issues and leave the explicit policy discussions for the end of the book. As an editor, he provided the kind of wisdom, guidance, and encouragement that is invaluable. Pamela Marshall improved the manuscript with her skillful and thorough copyediting. Where the language is faulty, the responsibility is mine.

Peggy Magnan helped immeasurably by typing the first draft of this book. Brian Egleston assisted greatly by helping type in his spare time when some crucial revisions were required.

Like most first books, this book was written in nooks and crannies of time while I was engaged in other studies and working full-time. This book never would have come into being without Tim's tremendous support, his patience, and humor, and that of B. and J. It is dedicated to them.

EQUAL PARTNERS

Introduction

Cure the disease and kill the patient.

——Francis Bacon

A WEEK after I graduated with honors from Harvard Medical School, I was in the neurological intensive care unit, having bled into my brain. This book travels through the year and a half that followed during which I was both a doctor and a patient. Being suddenly and seriously ill after years spent training to be a physician shed a harsh light on the health care doctors now provide in the United States. I learned quickly that, in the American health care system, patients all too often occupy the bottom rung of the ladder, with their legs tied to prevent them from climbing.

Physicians incompletely informing patients about treatment options is only one example of this. Doctors give all sorts of reasons for not honestly and fully apprising patients and their families, whether about the side effects of medications or the complications they may have from surgery. Some physicians do not understand how patients can be equal partners when patients know less about microbiology, physiology, and pharmacology. It does not occur to them that they know less than patients about what disease symptoms are like, how to live with chronic illness or medical treatments, how to survive acute life-threatening illnesses or injuries, how disease affects work and families, what values patients weigh in making choices, and many other aspects of living with illness and acute chronic conditions.

Some doctors contend that telling patients about potential side effects of care will make patients more likely either to refuse treatment or, if they accept treatment, to experience side effects. But studies have repeatedly demonstrated the opposite. When physicians share information with patients about their care, patients are more likely to follow physicians' recommendations. Furthermore, when physicians involve patients in decision making, the health of patients improves substantially. Patients' symptoms decrease, and laboratory tests of their health show improvement.

Physicians who want to treat patients as equal partners are frustrated by our health care system. Sharing information and decision making with patients takes time. Yet many health plans that will pay for nearly limitless medical technology (unnecessary as well as needed) will not pay for doctors and patients to talk together. In one health maintenance organization with a reputation for being among the better plans in Boston, physicians are allotted only twelve minutes with each patient. Twelve minutes is nowhere near enough time to learn how a patient with complex medical problems is doing, to examine him, and to discuss options for care together. Yet to cut labor costs, the administrators tried to reduce visits to ten minutes. Only a threatened strike by the physicians prevented the cut.

Partnerships depend on continuity. Yet doctor-patient relationships are repeatedly severed in our country because patients' health insurance is usually linked to their employment. When patients change employers or employers change the plans they offer, patients are often forced to change physicians. Physicians cannot fix this situation merely by agreeing to provide care under all health plans because plans limit the physi-

cians with whom they will contract. Patients with the greatest
health care needs are the most vulnerable to losing their physicians because some plans refuse to contract with doctors who
care primarily for patients with serious health conditions.

This book is about changes in health care that are simple yet
radical. Not radical in a political sense. The changes — ones that
would help place patients on an equal footing with doctors —
are about neither conservative nor liberal ideology. They are
radical because they require fundamental change. Power over
patients' lives would be returned to patients. As one step, doctors would be trained and allowed time to share understanding
and decision making with patients.

Because this book critiques the current health care system, one in which I continue to work and receive care, it has
been a hard book to write. Yet I was inevitably and painfully
brought back to writing it by the suffering of friends, family,
and strangers in our hands — in the hands of physicians.

The experiences of Bill, Sarah, Melissa, and John were
tragically typical. My father called to tell me about Bill. Bill had
just been diagnosed with stomach cancer. He went to the
hospital to have a highly specialized test performed, which
would determine whether the cancer involved all layers of his
stomach. That finding would reveal how long he had to live.
The oncologist who told him that the cancer had grown
through the entire stomach wall spent only five minutes with
him. Five minutes to tell him that he had a 10 to 20 percent
chance of survival and that to get that chance he would need to
have radical surgery. "Oh," the oncologist replied to Bill's
request for names of good surgeons, "anyone can do the surgery." He must have meant anyone with experience in that type
of cancer surgery. Bill had no idea how to find such a surgeon.
Then the oncologist was gone, and Bill was alone with his
problem.

Dr. Schultz told Sarah, "Sam will need to take antibiotics daily to prevent further infections, at least until he can have a test to see if there is reflux," referring to the backward flow of urine from the bladder to the kidneys. "If he does have reflux, he'll need to take daily antibiotics for at least a year." Sarah wanted to know the reasoning behind the physician's recommendations so she could decide what was best for her newborn son. She asked a number of questions in order to understand: "What does the test involve? . . . What happens if Sam does not take antibiotics? . . . Do daily antibiotics in a young infant affect the development of the immune system?" But Dr. Schultz would neither answer Sarah's questions directly nor respond honestly that he did not know the answers to some of the questions, that he was not sure anyone knew the answers to those questions. Instead, he tried to frighten Sarah into following his recommendations. Sarah tried again to get information: "How common is reflux in boys that have had just one urinary tract infection?" Her questions reflected her training in research. Dr. Schultz did not answer. He walked away, asking sarcastically, "Is Sam going to grow up to be an epidemiologist?" He was indignant about being pressed for information.

John had received treatment for infertility. He described a meeting he attended of fertility specialists at which doctors proposed putting three eggs in a dish with an anonymous donor's sperm and three with a husband's sperm. The "problem" for the doctors was that some couples wanted to give the husband's sperm a better chance of fertilizing the egg by exposing four eggs to the husband's sperm and only two eggs to the donor's sperm. The doctors' goal was to get the woman pregnant regardless of who was the biologic father. The couples' goal was to conceive a child that had both the husband and wife as biologic parents. Why, he wondered, couldn't the doctors understand the parents' point of view?

Melissa was herself a physician, receiving treatment for

infertility. On the day she ovulated she expected to try to conceive "the natural way," as she called it, at home in bed with her husband. She received a call from the clinic's nurse. The nurse stated matter-of-factly, "We discussed your case on rounds and agreed that it would be better for you to have intrauterine insemination, so you and your husband need to come in first thing tomorrow morning." Melissa knew what the words meant, but she did not know the reasoning behind the recommendation. Nor did the nurse. It never occurred to the doctor that Melissa would want to know why he was recommending artificial insemination, that Melissa and her husband might not want to conceive that way, or that Melissa and her husband would at least want to make an informed choice for themselves.

The disparity between Melissa's reaction to the call and her husband's was sad and telling. Her husband had been healthy his whole life, and it was his first contact with the health care system. The doctor's attitude shocked him. Melissa was discouraged but not surprised. She was a physician and had been a patient for decades because of a congenital condition that had required multiple surgeries. She had seen the exclusion of patients from decision making about their own lives, breakdowns in communication, and withholding of information many times before.

This book tells many patients' stories, including my own. (Patients' and doctors' names and identifying characteristics have been changed to protect their privacy.) In the body of the book, the stories are told with little commentary added. The details of our experiences are shared with the hope that they may help illuminate what it is like to be a patient in the U.S. health care system.

Newspapers tell stories of the singular wrongs some patients have suffered, such as deaths and disabilities that have resulted from malpractice or sexual harassment from abuse of power. This book is not the story of exceptional transgressions. Rather it tells stories of doctors' daily denials that patients are equals and of routine actions that regularly cause patients' care to suffer. The care of patients is habitually impoverished when patients' descriptions of their experiences are ignored, when doctors discourage patients from making decisions about their own care, when hospitals ignore patients' needs in everything from discharge routines to spring cleaning schedules, when patients' families are treated as invisible, and when health insurance provides doctors and patients with less and less time to talk to each other. Many of the insults are small — doctors not giving local anesthesia for temporarily painful procedures or nurses not calling a doctor when a hospitalized patient grows sicker and asks to be seen — but taken together, these regular wrongs are a stronger indictment of our current system than the less frequent acts of malpractice or rare acts of malevolence.

Writing about my own experiences was difficult. I have written about them not because I believe they are important in and of themselves — they are not — but because studies have shown that they are typical of what many patients experience. The goal of the body of the book is to give life to the studies that describe the problems patients face in our present health care system. Some of the statistics contained in these studies are discussed in the last chapter. The last chapter also explores how we could begin to transform health care.

As I wrote this book, Leslie Heafitz warned Harvard Medical School alumni about the position of patients in the United States. A doctor who had had cancer, she told other physicians, "Someday, every single one of you, sooner or later, will become a patient. And I dare say, you will not particularly like being on the other side of the fence." One week after graduating from medical school, I had begun to understand why.

CHAPTER ONE

Seized

IN JUNE 1989, I graduated from both Harvard Medical School and the Kennedy School of Government. My ten-month-old son could not figure out what all the fuss was about. Why was I dressed up in a black robe and why was Tim taking all these photographs before breakfast? I had wanted to bring Ben to graduation, but the rain was pouring. Ben went to day care, and we went to sit through hours of speeches under umbrellas, torrents of rain coming down. Still, it was a joyous time.

I had taken a circuitous path to medical school. Immediately after college, I went to Tanzania as a Peace Corps volunteer to train village cooperative members, schoolchildren, and farmers in how to raise fish.

Tanzania was the fourth-poorest country in the world, and malnutrition was, tragically, common. Many infectious diseases were endemic. Fish farming could potentially provide an important source of protein to the poor.

When Mdoe developed chronic malaria the year before I met him, he could no longer work. He could no longer grow corn or fish. His children grew hungry. Mdoe was too ill to repair the thatch on his hut. The roof let the rains in, and his family became sick.

The rural hospital that served the village where Mdoe and I lived had few medical supplies. The nurses would sit for hours crumpling pieces of white notebook paper until they became soft enough to be used as cotton balls. As I sat with them crumpling paper and worrying about how to help Mdoe's family, I began to think about becoming a doctor.

After attending medical school, I planned to return to work in developing countries. Knowing something about life's unexpected turns, I would routinely add to my plans the phrase "God and health willing." But the phrase had more rhythm than meaning to me then.

Eight years had passed since I had worked in Tanzania when, after the graduation ceremony, my family went for a sentimental dinner. The setting was elegant, or so it seemed. Any setting with no high chair at the table and no food on my clothes or the floor might have seemed elegant to me. We were all ecstatic. My parents toasted with champagne. I had never been a prizewinner before, and graduation had brought prizes from both Harvard Medical School and the Kennedy School of Government for work I had done in international health. It seemed that day that the world was giving prizes just for caring for other people. We do not have many photographs of the evening, but the joy is captured permanently in my heart, tinged only by the hindsight of knowing what would come afterward.

The week after graduation, Tim, Ben, and I set off for Amherst to visit my friend Ann and her family. Ann had been one of my closest college friends. After college, she had gone to work in Mali, in Saharan Africa. We had been close in every way except miles since college. This would be our only chance to see each other before the long haul of internship, when a day off would be a luxury, and a weekend off would come only a few times a year. Despite a headache, I stayed up late talking outside in the cool early summer breeze and then warming up in the kitchen with Tim, Ann, her husband, Ed, and their son, Jake. Ben slept in Tim's arms and Jake in Ann's. Other than our whispered conversation and the whistle of Ann's boiling tea kettle, the night had grown silent. At last we all went upstairs to bed in adjacent rooms. Tim and I crept into a small guest room where Ben's crib lay inches from our single bed. Tim moved an arm here, I bumped an elbow there, our knees hit as we tried to sleep side by side in the small bed. We whispered to each other in the darkness until we finally dozed off.

Hours later, I woke up in a large, sharply overlit room. The room was stifling hot; no windows were visible. Loud male voices called incomprehensibly to each other. My arms and legs were strapped down tightly to the hard slab beneath me. I was unable to move. I could see only the ceiling and the tops of the walls as two strangers kept passing by me, in and out of my field of vision. I began asking for Tim. The strangers did not respond.

As my thoughts began to clear, I tried to put together the few pieces of information I had. I had been moved by strangers to a foreign location. No other women were in sight. The men would not talk to me and had tied me down so I could not move. Not knowing where I was and what these men were doing terrified me, but more immediately I was frightened for Tim. What had they done to him? Only moments ago we had been nestled together safely in bed.

"Tim? . . . Tim? . . . Tim! . . . TIM!" My voice grew louder and more urgent when there was no response. The men continued to hustle about as if they had a plan. I cried out again for Tim, desperately worried about him, as I tried to figure out what type of place I was in.

After a long time, one of the strangers finally spoke: "He'll be back."

"Yeah, right," I thought, too frightened of the man to challenge him. If he wasn't conning me, why wouldn't he explain where I was or what was going on? I kept calling for Tim, thinking that the first job I had to do was get us back together.

"He can't hear you," said the stranger, trying to shut me up, peering down at me as I lay captive, still strapped at the ankles and wrists. The prolonged, terror-filled silence continued.

At last, Tim came within sight. Holding my hand, he explained that we were in a hospital. When we had arrived, he had been told he had to leave me to go to admitting to sign in. The hospital's signals were clear: the first emergency was getting information about our health insurance. Afterward, he was told to follow a procedure routinely painful for patients and family members and often unnecessary; he had to wait outside. Finally, after my persistent confused cries, he was allowed in. Once at my side in the emergency room, in the middle of the night, he was the first person to tell me that I had had a seizure and had been brought to the local hospital by ambulance.

More than a year later, when the pain had partially abated, we sat on a futon by the window in our apartment, and he told me the details of what had happened.

All of a sudden I had started pushing Tim in the back. He rolled over to see what I was doing, and it was obvious that I was having a seizure. My eyes were rolled up. My teeth were clenched. He rolled me onto my side and shouted for Ed and Ann to get an ambulance.

Ann spoke softly but urgently into the phone: "I'm at thirteen Dogwood Street, and we need an ambulance."

"What's going on?"

"We need an ambulance," she repeated, trying to get one quickly, not wanting to waste time with a long conversation.

"Well, describe what's happening," the operator replied, enunciating each word slowly, purposefully, and with some frustration.

Initially, Ann tried to explain. Then, exasperated, she settled on "Her husband's a doctor, and he says that we need an ambulance."

When the emergency medical technicians finally arrived, Tim introduced himself and explained the situation rapidly: "Tim Brewer. I'm her husband, a doctor. She'd just fallen asleep when she had a tonic clonic seizure."

As they half listened, the EMTs tried to move me without explaining to me who they were. Post-ictal, experiencing the short-lived but profound confusion that can follow a generalized seizure, I had no idea what was going on. Unaware of what had happened and that an ambulance had been called, terrified of these strangers who were taking me away, I started trying to fight them off.

"What drugs is she taking?" the EMTs asked repeatedly, believing neither Tim's account of the seizure nor his straightforward response: "None."

Tim went on to explain that the EMTs neither told me what they were going to do nor tried to reassure me. The EMTs continued to talk only to him. Throughout the entire episode, from strapping me to a stretcher through the ambulance ride to the hospital, I was treated as a drug addict and Tim as guilty by association.

While I held hands with Tim in the emergency room, the obvious fact that I was the patient and not the doctor nearly eluded me. Silently, I began to tick off the routine steps for handling an adult with her first seizure. My doctors would need to rule out a tumor, a bleed, or some other cause of a focal lesion in my brain. I anticipated the CAT scan, which was the next step, before the orderlies began to wheel my stretcher to the radiology suite.

Only when the emergency room doctor approached me after the brain scan and told me he would need to do a second scan, with contrast, did the reality of my situation begin to sink in. He did not give any reasons for the second CAT scan, but his evasiveness only confirmed what was frighteningly obvious to me.

"You found something wrong?"

"Yes, we found a space-occupying lesion. We don't know what it is, so we'd like to take a look at it with contrast."

"The contrast will help you tell if it's cancer."

He nodded his head in silent assent.

After the second CAT scan was performed, the doctors told Tim they thought I had bled into my brain, but they could not be sure without further testing. They explained that their hospital did not have the facilities to deal with an intracranial bleed. They recommended that I be transferred to a major medical center like Regional that had a Magnetic Resonance Imager to clarify what was wrong in my brain as well as a neurological intensive care unit where I could be treated by a neurosurgical staff if anything went wrong. Even though I was by now alert and coherent, the post-ictal confusion having long since dissipated, the doctor reviewed the different hospitals to which I could be transferred with Tim alone.

Tim went to find a hospital pay phone. He stood looking for change, asking himself whether he should wish my parents a happy thirty-fifth wedding anniversary before breaking the news.

My father picked up the phone groggily, awakened from a deep sleep. "Is something wrong, Tim?"

"Everything's okay," he said, hoping to sound casual. "Jody just had a seizure, and I wanted to see if I could get Jim Griffin's phone number." The two statements were incongruous. If everything was okay, why was he calling at 2:00 A.M. for the phone number of a neurologist?

"Should we come up tonight?" my father asked immediately. He was worried. It was not just the seizure. It was something in Tim's usually unflappable voice that frightened him.

Over and over again my mother asked Tim questions to which he didn't yet know the answers. In the end, Tim explained that the doctors thought I had bled into my brain.

After the call, my father lay anxiously awake, and my mother frantically made arrangements for a 7:00 A.M. flight. Tim and I went by ambulance to the Regional Medical Center.

More sobering than the two-and-a-half-hour ambulance ride, strapped down next to resuscitation equipment, was the two-and-a-half-minute trip to my bed in the neurologic intensive care unit. On the way, we passed people in the hall who had recently undergone neurosurgery: a man strapped into his wheelchair because he could no longer support the weight of his own body; a woman with a bandaged head who had drooled from her mouth, which she could no longer control; and, the most mobile of all, a young man dragging a paralyzed arm and leg behind him as he walked. They were all on the recovery ward.

As what I might have to face was being transformed into reality before my eyes, I held on to a peculiar belief nurtured in medical school that one can and should talk oneself out of fear of disease, disability, treatments, and death. I once would have argued that it is how people deal with fears we all experience that separates out those who are courageous. I still believe that, but I now know more about the cost of courage, the fact that it can be as maladaptive at times as it is adaptive at others.

The patients on the ward were doing far better than those in the intensive care unit, the majority of whom still had tubes to help them breathe, eat, and collect their urine. Tim read the many plaques on the wall that honored the chief of neurosurgery. I didn't notice them as I was being wheeled past on a gurney. Tim and I were beginning to walk in different shoes; the ripped foam patient slippers were beginning to fit my feet that night, though I would still fight against them. Only a week had passed since graduation.

Soon after we arrived at my room, a doctor told Tim that he should go to sleep. It was the middle of the night, and Tim was in a strange city with no transportation and no place to stay. He wandered the hospital until he found an empty waiting room and fell asleep on the vinyl couches to the smell of cleaning fluid and the tune of the buzzing fluorescent lights. The doctor did not tell Tim where he might go to sleep. The omission was small but sadly symptomatic of how commonly our health care system ignores both small and large obstacles faced by patients' families.

The next morning, I was wheeled to the Magnetic Resonance Imager and given a little red ball to hold between my fingers and squeeze if anything went wrong. Magnetic Resonance Imaging is one of the latest technologies for looking inside the human body. The machine transforms electromagnetic signals into a detailed picture of the inside of the human body and brain. MRIs are a cross between a physicist's idea of heaven and a claustrophobic's idea of hell. They make a casket look roomy. The patient is rolled on a dolly into the bowels of the machine, its hard casing centimeters away from the patient's nose and ears. There is no room to move either arms or legs. Isolated from technicians and physicians in a soundproof room, the patient can communicate only by means of the ball.

The method works as long as the patient does not lose consciousness. As magnetic fields build up, the machine sounds like a cold metal radiator as it fills with steam. Still, after a night spent in ambulances, an emergency room, and an intensive care unit, being repeatedly prodded and examined, I fell asleep in the isolation of the MRI.

Afterward, waiting for the verdict of whether or not I had brain cancer was like waiting for a sentencing that would determine the course of the rest of my life. I thought about how this process was as routine for the radiologists as brushing their teeth. There would first be a dicussion about all the possible causes of the seizure, some teaching and grilling of medical students or residents, and then a "reading" of what the X ray probably showed, with a lengthy description of alternative diagnoses. The discussion might include such comments as "this is an interesting case" or "this is a sad case," but it would not cause more pause than a shake of the head or a slightly prolonged sigh.

My parents arrived shortly before we were due to hear the MRI results. My mother's thoughts darted back and forth with her eyes. She was searching for curtains so we could talk as a family, at least out of sight if not out of earshot of strangers. She tried to avoid both staring at the postoperative woman in the next bed and thinking about what her daughter would go through if surgery was necessary.

My mother had worried about whether or not Tim and I would want her and my father to fly up but she knew she needed to be there, to see things firsthand. After arriving, my father also worried about his role as the parent of an adult. He felt like the "inner circle" was supposed to be patient and doctor, then the next circle included the patient's spouse. Somehow he felt parents lay outside both circles. Many parents have questions about their roles as parents of a sick child. Their questions usually go unrecognized in our health care system; my parents' did.

The afternoon of the MRI, Dr. Jackson, the senior neuro-surgeon on call, came to see me. He explained that the MRI showed what he thought was a vascular malformation or tu-mor, not cancer as far as he could tell. The hemangioma, or cluster of abnormal blood vessels, had bled into my brain, and the bleeding had caused a seizure. He recommended that the hemangioma be surgically removed. He was happy either to do the surgery himself or to refer us to a surgeon near our home.

The recommendation of brain surgery made Tim call Boston for the advice of physicians he knew. The neurologist he phoned said we should return to Boston to get a second opinion and, if we decided to go ahead with the surgery, have it done close to home.

Lying in my hospital bed, separated from Ben and Tim, I worried about how the bleed would affect my ability to contribute both at home and at work, although I had no idea how profoundly the injury would change the simple elements of my daily life. During those first days and weeks, I asked each doctor who cared for me what it meant to live with seizures. None answered. No one talked with me about how my life would change or told me what was still safe to do and what wasn't or even mentioned that legally I had to stop driving until I was seizure-free for six months.

There are many diseases that health care workers cannot cure but that they can help patients live with. In each case, it would make such a difference if at least one physician did individual counseling at the time of the diagnosis and then again as changes occurred in the patient's condition or treatments available. What a difference it would make if physicians would ask patients such questions as "What do you like to do?" or "How do you usually spend your time?"; discuss how those activities will be affected by the medical problem and treatment options; and develop a plan together with the patient.

If my aunt and cousin had been counseled well when they both had seizures from cancer metastasizing to their brains, then I might have thought that the omission was because I was a doctor. If I did not go on as a physician to witness the same vacuum created for many other patients and their families when they developed seizures, then I would have thought the omissions were rare.

CHAPTER TWO

Choosing Without Knowing

O NCE I GOT HOME from the hospital, it was evident how little I could do. During the first day home, I had strength for only a few hours of sitting. Tim spent the day at work, Ben at day care, and I in bed or crawling to the kitchen.

We had been sent back to Boston with no one in charge of my care. Dr. Jackson had recommended we call a Dr. Manson. When we did call the first day, we found out that Dr. Manson would not be able to see us for two weeks.

My first night home, Tim woke up at 4:00 A.M. I was sitting up crying in bed; I had the worst headache I had ever had, a symptom often signaling blood cells on the brain from a severe infection or hemorrhage. My eyes couldn't see past the thick fog the pain created; even my thoughts could not penetrate its intensity. For the first time, Tim felt scared. He had rarely seen me cry and as a physician he knew that the headaches to worry most about are the ones that wake patients in the middle of the night. Most stress headaches happen during the daytime, when people are awake and aware of their stress. Headaches that occur when people sleep are the ones that make physicians worry about tumors or other causes of increased pressure inside the skull, pressure that is exacerbated by lying down. As I pleaded for pain relief, Tim grew anxious and called Sinai Hospital, where he worked. "Can you please page the neurologist on call?"

Most patients who have been discharged from a distant hospital without a doctor to care for them cannot just call up a local hospital and page a specialist. They end up going by car or ambulance to an emergency room. When they arrive in the emergency room, there is a long wait to be seen, followed by another long wait while the hospital staff searches for information. When neither a doctor who has cared for the patient nor medical records can be found, tests are often repeated, treatments are chosen in partial ignorance, time is lost, hundreds to thousands of dollars are wasted, and the quality of the care suffers along with the patient. Over and over again.

We sat in the dark waiting. Tim had tried to turn on the light before phoning but I had screamed in pain — another bad sign. Patients who have had bleeds onto the surface of their brains can be markedly photophobic. The only light in the room was from the glowing numbers on the phone.

Tim drove to Sinai to get medicine that the neurologist on call prescribed after asking enough questions to rule out a life-threatening new bleed. I sat huddled in our darkened bedroom, hoping that Lamaze breathing might somehow ease the pain that, unlike labor contractions, was constant and unabating. Ben stirred and cried in the next room. Although our bedroom door was shut, our apartment was too small for the sound of my cries, Tim's phone call, and his departure for the hospital not to have woken Ben.

The headaches continued to wake me up every night until I began sleeping sitting up as I had in the hospital. This reduced the pressure from fluid on top of a tumor or abnormal blood vessels in my brain. After sleepless nights, we spent the days making calls to find a neurologist who was recommended, not overbooked, and not on summer vacation who would see us. I worried about how the change in my health burdened Tim and how it might affect his feelings toward me. Tim reminds me now that I kept asking him, "How are you doing dealing with it all? . . . Are you feeling okay about things?"

"I'm doing fine. You're the one that has to go through this," he would respond. But I knew that was not true. We were both going through it.

Dr. Jackson was a wonderful, caring physician. I can imagine how inadequate follow-up care was arranged. Dr. Jackson may have called Dr. Manson and explained my case to him. The residents knew that the "referral had been made." It was written on the appropriate line on the discharge papers, but no one knew how long it would take to get an appointment. That's a common omission in discharges — one that again reflects that discharges are done from the doctor's point of view, not the patient's or family's.

Not having a doctor was only one part of our problem. The fact that the physicians in charge did not discuss with either Tim or me prevention of and response to the headaches and the possibility of ongoing bleeding was another. After caring for the hemorrhage without discussion in the hospital, the doctors did not have or spend the time to think that that care would fall on us upon discharge.

Despite his being a physician, the first days home were the hardest for Tim because he felt "nobody was in control," "nobody was watching out." How much harder it must be daily for the thousands of families with no medical background who are left without a primary physician, having been dropped down the crevices in our health care system.

From a doctor's vantage point, the "discharge planning" had all been so routine: the patient got sick while she was traveling. Once she is stabilized, does the patient wish to continue her care where she is now or return home for "definitive care"? If she's going to return home, we will just need to give her a referral for follow-up care.

Referrals for follow-up care are a routine part of the majority of discharge planning. In the busy life of residents, discharge planning is almost a necessary evil. It gets squeezed in between more immediate demands in the hospital.

Hospital routines regularly ignore the majority of discharge needs patients and their families have. Studies have highlighted that discharge planning is one of the most problematic areas of in-patient care.

Tim brought home the *New England Journal of Medicine* after work and left it on the kitchen table. The journal is among the most respected for publishing new findings from well-conducted medical research. On the cover was an article entitled "Pattern of Malformations in the Children of Women Treated with Carbamezipine During Pregnancy."

Carbamezipine is the generic name for the anticonvulsant Tegretol, which I would be taking. Before the article was published, specialists had been confident that Tegretol was a safe — and probably the only safe — anticonvulsant to take during pregnancy. I started to cry as I watched Ben happily cruise around the kitchen in his seat on wheels. Tim and I were ready for a second child.

Over time, new research results are critically reviewed by the scientific community. Findings may be reversed as errors in the research methodology are revealed. But Tim and I needed to decide soon. Our thinking and that of the doctors who cared for me was significantly affected by that article, biased as it might have been by factors including the pressure on academic researchers to publish rapidly and the greater willingness of journals to print "positive findings." I wondered if most medical

authors realized that how they describe tentative findings immediately and dramatically affects people's lives.

I pored over the details of the *New England Journal of
Medicine* article again and again, trying to figure out if the study
had been well conducted. If the conclusions were right,
Tegretol was a very dangerous drug to take during pregnancy.
Some of the methodology seemed weak and some of the conclusions questionable, but the article did not provide enough of
the original data to be sure.

By the time we were able to see Dr. Manson, two concerns had
emerged: trying to get off anticonvulsants so Tim and I could
safely have another child and trying to prevent seizures so we
could return to work overseas.

My parents had raised me to believe that work involved
trying to make a difference in other people's lives. Over a half
dozen years, at first working with homeless people living in the
streets of New York, I had grown committed to working on
health care for those who had little or none. The summer after
starting medical school, I went into the refugee camps in southern Mexico. War and government repression had forced more
than a million Guatemalans to flee their homes and be displaced
within their own country or become refugees in other countries, principally Mexico. Meeting health care workers from
Guatemala touched me profoundly. The national university
there had a rural health program. Eight people working in rural
health care were killed or disappeared in one summer alone.
Yet, despite the dangers, Guatemalan health care workers continued to work with poor underserved communities.

Throughout medical school, I went down to the refugee
camps and to Guatemala again and again on different projects. I
began to work to support projects that would help train Guatemalan refugee health care workers and provide services to rural

Mexicans. For our honeymoon, Tim and I went to the Albert Schweitzer Hospital in Gabon, West Africa, to provide medical care. We planned as a family to work abroad as well as in the United States. Now the possibility of further bleeds in my brain and unpredictable seizures also threatened our working in remote areas where there was little health care.

Dr. Manson squeezed us in on a Sunday afternoon. He was so busy that it had taken two weeks to find time even on a Sunday. When he returned our first phone call after ten at night, we were already in bed, and he was still seeing patients in the hospital. His commitment to long hours was matched by his secretary's; she was in the office that Sunday afternoon to greet us as if it were any Monday morning.

Dr. Manson came out from behind his desk to shake our hands. Then he sat back down, white-haired and weary. For the first several minutes I could not take my eyes off his hands. Was there a mild tremor, or was he just tired and jittery from too much caffeine that afternoon? The vascular tumor lay fractions of an inch from the part of the brain that controls one's ability to move one's left side.

Tim's eyes wandered over Dr. Manson's bookcase and stopped on a textbook as large as the textbooks that detail all of adult medicine. This textbook, however, was entirely devoted to tumors of the third ventricle, one small part of the brain.

In medicine, the term *tumor* technically means "a space-occupying lesion" or anything that takes up space where it is not supposed to be; the term does not refer only to cancer. What was in my brain was often referred to as a tumor of malformed blood vessels.

Before our first meeting with Dr. Manson, Tim and I had written out a list of questions so that we would not forget what to ask in the limited time physicians usually had.

Does surgery increase or decrease the risk of seizures?

Is the effect of the surgical scar or the hemangioma worse?

What is the risk of more bleeds?

Does surgery make your health more predictable than if the hemangioma was there and you could still have a bleed?

If this is how we, as doctors, felt going into a doctor's office — that it was necessary to write our questions out — how must other patients feel?

Beside the list of carefully written questions we planned to write the answers. That way, if discussing the surgery in the office was overwhelming, in the quiet of home we would know what the answers had been. We soon learned that it would be hard to fill an article let alone a textbook with what was known about the treatment of cavernous hemangiomas. After our discussions, Dr. Manson recommended surgery.

Because Dr. Manson could not operate for two months, and to get one more opinion before brain surgery, we went to see Dr. Barrows, a second neurosurgeon, who had been recommended to us. As Dr. Barrows spoke to us in his office, Tim fiddled with the beads on a child's toy from the waiting area. After reviewing my medical history and X rays, Dr. Barrows concluded, "I think you should have the lesion removed. . . . It's not located near anything important in your brain since you're not left-handed. That's unless you want to be a concert pianist," he added with a smile.

For some left-handed people the right side of the brain is dominant in their abilities to speak, comprehend, and write. These abilities are concentrated in the part of the brain where the tumor lay. In right-handed people, the same part of the brain can affect fine musical abilities (of which I had never demonstrated any).

So important is it to know the dominant hemisphere with certainty that brain surgery for epilepsy is sometimes done under local anesthesia. With the patient awake, the nerve cells can be stimulated and the function of each small area of the brain mapped. But Dr. Barrows did not want to do the operation without general anesthesia. My tumor was probably a hemangioma with only small amounts of blood in it, but no one knew for sure. Other vascular malformations can bleed uncontrollably. Dr. Barrows explained that if something went wrong during surgery, "it's easier to respond if the patient is under general anesthesia." That was the sanitized way of saying that if the patient begins to die, doctors have a better chance of saving him than if the patient is under only local anesthesia. With general anesthesia, there is a tube connected to the patient's lungs with which the anesthesiologist is aleady helping the patient breathe.

Dr. Barrows couldn't say what effect the surgery would have on my seizures in the short run. "Most people say removing hemangiomas and other vascular malformations will reduce seizures, but I'm just not sure. . . . Removing the lesion will reduce seizures, but the surgical scar left behind could increase them."

Tim was relieved that Dr. Barrows, whose reputation as a neurosurgeon was superb, could perform the surgery soon. He was worried about waiting as my headaches persisted. He spent nights wondering if I were bleeding again in my head. Although Dr. Manson's prediction that the bleeds were unlikely to be life-threatening was somewhat reassuring, it was not reassuring enough.

Medicine is often portrayed as providing a near perfect understanding of — if not perfect solutions to — problems. In reality, often the best we have to offer as physicians is honesty about the limitations of our knowledge and help responding to the many uncertainties patients face.

Mehran, a patient I had seen during medical school, had been forced to make a far graver choice based on little information. At forty, he had spent more than twenty years of his life working as a truck driver to support his five children. He had always dreamed of returning to his home in Isfahan and writing poetry. Now, he had metastatic melanoma. He was desperately torn between returning to his childhood home while he still felt well and gambling on an experimental new therapy that had the chance of offering a cure if it worked. If it failed, the treatment would steal his remaining healthy months. His wife kept pressing for more information on the success of the new treatment. All any of the doctors could say was "We don't know. We won't know for three to five years, when preliminary research is done." By then it would be too late. Still, it mattered to Mehran that physicians honestly shared their uncertainty.

Tim and I had spoken to brain surgeons at three different hospitals. The doctors' level of uncertainty and disagreement was striking, though not uncommon in health care. Dr. Jackson advised us that what he believed was an arteriovenous malformation could bleed again at unpredictable times, and suggested that surgery would significantly lower the risk of seizures by preventing subsequent bleeding into my brain. Dr. Manson felt the tumor was a hemangioma and recommended surgery to decrease the chance of further seizures caused by the presence of the tumor. Dr. Barrows thought that, although what he saw on the MRI was probably a hemangioma, no one could be sure without operating. Surgery was important to make sure it was not cancer.

The neurosurgeons did all agree on one thing: whatever it was should be removed. They also agreed that the surgery would be brief, probably an hour and a half or less from start to finish, and that it would not pose any risk of harming my skills; the lesion was not near anything of consequence in my brain. (I was starting to appreciate all the unused parts of our brains our elementary school teachers tried to chastise us into using as we grew up.)

The decision seemed clear. Everyone had recommended surgery. Their reasons varied, but mine seemed clear. First, I wanted to do everything I could to get off anticonvulsants and have a safe pregnancy. I knew that I would not be able to live with myself if I gave birth to a child with congenital anomalies and had not done everything in my power to avoid them. After tallying all the votes, the majority opinion was that the best chance of avoiding anticonvulsants during pregnancy was through surgery. Second, the safest way to continue to work in developing countries was to be free of the risk of recurrent bleeds. The best decision for me might not have been the best decision for someone who did not want to become pregnant and would never live far from a major medical center.

The sooner the better. I was anxious to return to work and felt pressure from Renee, the chief resident who would supervise my program, to begin my internship as soon as possible. Headaches still made the nights as difficult as low blood pressure did the days. No one wanted to change my anticonvulsant, despite the side effects, until after the surgery.

Dr. Barrows would be able to operate in a week and a half. Dr. Manson would not be able to do so for two months. Each week seemed like a year of waiting, so Tim and I decided to have Dr. Barrows do the surgery. Both surgeons had excellent reputations, even if Dr. Barrows was somewhat less well known internationally. It was supposed to be such a simple operation.

My parents' pain was no less intense than my own, and their distance from the decision making made their anguish more profound. Maybe one of them had the notion first or maybe my parents each came up with it independently, but the image stuck to them both like burs to a dog: "What if the surgeon's scalpel slipped?" my father said in a strained, quiet voice. "If he slips, he could cut out half of her ability to think or do anything else. God!" That was it. In their minds, anything could happen.

Although I tried to reassure them both, repeating the surgeons' assurances that the surgery was very minor for brain surgery, my questions about left-handedness undermined my efforts to reassure. I questioned my mother several times: "Was I ever left-handed as a child?" "Did you have to encourage me to be right-handed?" "Are you sure I wasn't a lefty and then pushed to switch?" Too much rested on an accurate answer. If I had always been right-handed, then operating on the part of my brain where the abnormal blood vessels lay posed little threat to future functionality.

My father had taught methods of rational decision making to graduate students. He tried to reason a decision by returning to those methods. He made up an elaborate decision tree of all the choices and risks and benefits from different courses of action. But it only ignited his anger at neurosurgeons, at what in his eyes was their abysmal ignorance. They were all proposing surgery, but none could answer the basic questions on which such a decision would rationally be based. How likely is the tumor to be something other than a hemangioma? How likely is the surgery to prevent future seizures? The list went on. The only question the surgeons would all answer similarly was that the risks of the surgery were low and that the operation was simple and would be brief. So, in their eyes it was worth it, even if the magnitude of the benefits was unknown.

My father began to crack the kinds of jokes about neurosurgeons, chipping away at their pedestal, that had been made about space scientists after the crash of the *Challenger*. Only my own crash would silence the jokes.

I tried to explain to my father that while I would love to have a long and meaningful life, a meaningful life was more important to me than a long one. As I was growing up, my mother often told me the story of a man who was so afraid of dying that he would never go out and do anything. He grew to a very old age and then realized that he had never lived. She recounted the story so often that I grew up much more afraid of that kind of life — of never taking risks, never daring to love, never caring about the world, never trying to change things for the better — than of the accidental or medical causes of death beyond one's control. She taught me that courage did not mean having no fear. Courage meant living according to one's beliefs. Courage meant acting on the belief that each of us can make a difference in the world.

A week before the surgery, a card from Mrs. Rivers arrived. She wrote gently, "You have not been the luckiest person." I laughed because despite everything, I still felt extremely lucky. I had the most loving husband, with whom I could share laughter, tears, joys, and fears. Ben brought an indescribable amount of joy into our lives. My parents and my brother shared their wisdom and their sense of the sublime and ridiculous while giving me boundless love. My family gave me the tremendous gift of knowing that the love and friendship we give away comes back to us many times over. I had had twenty-nine wonderful years full of learning and friendship, working in situations as different as African villages with schoolchildren and New York City parks with the homeless. My friends had stood by me through all of life's ups and downs.

Yes, I wanted to live and love for another fifty years, to watch Ben grow older with Tim, to spend much more time with my family and friends. Yes, I wanted to work for another fifty years and make a difference in the world. But whatever happened, I could not have more to be grateful for.

I thought I knew what I was in for. I had been sick before, hospitalized before, even had life-threatening malaria before, and I was a physician. But I hadn't a clue. It was the courage of someone who doesn't know what she is about to face.

CHAPTER THREE

Where Patients Are Placed

Nothing places a thing so intensely in the
memory as the wish to forget it.

—*Montaigne*

Dr. Heymann is a 29 year old right-handed woman who was in
excellent health until one week ago about midnight she had a
major motor seizure. . . . Her MRI shows a discrete circular
lesion a little over 1 cm in diameter in the superior temporal
gyrus on the right side. There is a question of a little blood in
that area. This may be a small angiomatous malformation or
perhaps a small tumor which has bled. At any rate, because of
its superficial location in the nondominant hemisphere I think
clearly the best thing to do is to have the lesion excised.

—Thomas Barrows, M.D.

ON JULY 6, Tim drove me to the hospital. We sat in the
admitting area and held on to each other as we waited for the
process to begin. The waiting room had the same new crim-
son and aquamarine walls, carpeting, and furniture as every

hospital facility in Boston that had been newly built or reno-
vated in the last five years. There must have been a study
calling the colors calming.

The waiting room was oddly empty — no patients, no
staff — and odorless. After twenty minutes alone, nestled in
each other's arms in silence, we were called. That was the
last time I'd ever feel complete and naive trust in a hospital
admission.

The admissions clerk handed us forms to fill out. Name.
Address. Person to notify in case of emergency. Insurance.
Group number. Subscriber name. Relationship. Guarantor if
insurance won't pay. Signatures were required to consent to
any and all procedures: "Permission is given to the University
Hospital, Inc., and its physicians, employees, agents and servants for the performance of any diagnostic examination, treatment, biopsy, transfusion and/or surgical procedure, and for
the administration of any anesthetic that may be deemed advisable in the course of this hospital admission."

"Informed consent" is legally required. Patients are to be
told about each medication given or procedure performed for
diagnosis and treatment, about the risks and benefits, and about
what alternatives could be considered. The law requires that
consent be voluntary, given under no duress. Unfortunately,
what commonly occurs is the universal "uninformed acknowledgment," that anyone may perform "any diagnostic examination,
treatment, biopsy, transfusion and/or surgical procedure," in
which what will happen to the patient is unspecified, the risks,
benefits, and alternatives not even touched on. Such "consent" is
only voluntary in the most limited sense. The choice is: sign here
or we will not admit you.

Tim was asked to sign as the insurance policyholder and as
someone committed to pay the bills if I died. All requirements,
promises of payment, and submissions fulfilled, we were sent

upstairs. The institutionalization began. The hospital bracelet went on, the street clothes were stripped off in a hospital room with no decorations and no personal artifacts on a ward filled with patients wearing identical gowns and bracelets.

Dr. Barrows had arranged for me to be admitted the day before surgery for preoperative testing. He scheduled a preoperative arteriogram to make sure that the abnormal blood vessels were veins and not arteries. Arteries, which contain blood at a higher pressure than veins, present a much greater danger of life-threatening bleeds. In preparation for the arteriogram, a resident positioned me on a table in the radiology suite next to the television-sized screen, which would show the inside of my head. Tim was asked to leave as the resident tried unsuccessfully to get a large bore needle into my groin.

Outside, another resident talked to Tim about how tumors are often localized for brain surgery. A "halo" is used. A halo is headgear, more reminiscent of Frankenstein than of Gabriel, which is bolted with screws to a patient's skull so that it will not move. "Pointers" are then positioned using a CAT scan to mark where the tumor is, so that there will be no doubt where the surgeons should cut. But hemangiomas like mine do not show up as well on a CAT scan as on an MRI, and the metal halos routinely used in CAT scans could not be placed in the magnetic field of the MRI machine. The radiologists were waiting for plastic halos, a relatively simple but potentially critical device to lack in a multimillion-dollar high-technology MRI suite.

In the absence of halos, surgeons rely on their reading of the MRI to localize the lesion. Although surgeons often repeat radiologic exams at their own hospital to confirm the findings before operating, Dr. Barrows did not feel it was necessary to run another MRI. He was certain that the map that the MRI from Regional Medical Center provided was all he needed.

* * *

The resident missed the artery in my groin four times. He had chosen not to use a local anesthetic, saying, "I can get this needle in on the first try. Local anesthesia would just mean sticking you twice instead of once." But when he was unable to insert the needle, he didn't stop to provide pain relief. A large bore needle is large enough for a catheter or plastic tube to be passed through its center, into the groin, up through the abdomen, through the chest, and into the brain, where it will release dye. The needles used for local anesthetic are tiny. Throughout his attempts I kept silent, except for reflexively gritting my teeth to the pain, understanding that everyone has to learn sometime. The fifth time, the more senior supervising physician insisted that the resident numb the area. After two more missed attempts by the resident, the senior physician placed the large bore needle on his first try. Living with unavoidable brief pain from needed procedures was not bad. But the unnecessary pain caused by the resident not giving local anesthetic provided me with another window onto doctor-patient relationships, and the thin soil of distance in which they were sustained.

After completing the arteriogram, the resident told me, "Don't move. We'll wheel you upstairs. You need to stay flat on your back for six hours so we can make sure where we went in with the needle doesn't bleed too much."

Being wheeled through the hallway was like putting my nose in a tub full of ammonia, so it was a relief to get back into the room. Within moments a nurse came by to ask me, "How's that leg?" Without waiting for an answer, as people do when they ask "How are you?" to someone passing in the street, she continued, "I'm going to wheel you into the hallway for a couple hours while they clean out your room. We're scrubbing all the rooms today." So began hours in the hall, unable to move amid the bustle, barely covered by a Johnny, which they frequently lifted to uncover and check my groin, required to use a bedpan, numbed by the stench of hospital-strength cleaning fluid.

I was okay in the hallway, although no one would have chosen the public physical exams or toileting, or the stench. But it made clear where patients are placed in the hospital hierarchy. It would have been just as easy for the hospital to organize care so that rooms were cleaned in between patients' admissions.

Back in the room, the evening visiting hours with Tim passed rapidly. When Tim left, I lay staring at the blank wall for hours, as many patients in that room had before me, wondering about surgery, trying to sleep but unused to sleeping alone, loneliness mirrored by the bare room. Intermittent sleep finally came, interrupted at first by the hall lights and noises, and by nurses coming to check vital signs, and then by a disoriented patient's screams and my roommate fighting the drugs she had been given.

The next morning, I counted the tiles on the ceiling a dozen times waiting for my family to come before the surgery. My parents arrived. I do not remember what we talked about. I just remember us all sitting together huddled on and around the hospital bed. Bruce, the physician's aide, came to explain what would follow in more detail than any physician ever would.

"When they are ready for you in the operating room," he began, "I'll be giving you a premedication. We give it to all surgical patients to help them relax. Then I'll take you down to the operating room. You probably won't remember much of the day because the medicine that makes you relax also makes most people forget everything that happens between the time when they get the medicine in their room and the time when they come to in the recovery room. Some people remember waking up in the recovery room, but others don't. After the surgery, we'll take you to the neurosurgical intensive care unit. The nurses gave you a tour?"

"Yes." The nurses had showed us what the unit looked like through the doorway.

We had seen all the patients in the intensive care unit from the door, their heads entirely covered with bandages, eyes and noses barely visible, some able to breathe on their own, others needing machines to breathe for them, tubes going in and coming out of every hole in their bodies, unable to eat on their own, unable to urinate on their own. No one was moving. They were not just the "not walking wounded" — they were not sitting and not talking.

Bruce went on to explain, "The surgery should last for only an hour and a half, and then Dr. Barrows can call Tim, and Tim can call your parents. Don't worry. It's a very straight-forward procedure; there won't be any problems." He was interrupted by an orderly who appeared at the door with a stretcher. Bruce injected a benzodiazepine into my intravenous line.

We tried to say cheerful good-byes as the medicine rap-idly began to take effect. Starting down the hall, I went back to counting the ceiling tiles, which were all I could see.

Not only was the surgery supposed to be short but Dr. Jackson, at Regional Medical Center, had said it was simple enough that "a third-year resident could perform it." At seven in the morning, as the preoperative medications began to gray the corners of the ceiling, which I could see from the stretcher, I was wheeled into the operating room.

It was almost two years before my father could talk with me about that day. He reopened the journal he filled the week of the surgery.

"Mom and I got up around four-thirty in the morning and

drove down to the hospital. I remember we saw you for about a half hour before they started to give you the series of sedatives. I remember them wheeling you down the hall to the operating area, and again your spirits were very good. There was something — an excruciating, sweet, proud, frightening feeling — about seeing you so brave and so upbeat going into something that was so frightening."

I remember trying to cheer my parents up but I also remember not being afraid, having the courage of a pilot who had studied war at the air force academy but never fought, at least never fought on the side that gets injured. It's frightening what a lack of perspective one can have even after medical training and working in hospital wards.

"Mom and I went home," Dad continued. "We sort of rambled around the house at first, not talking to each other or doing anything, trying not to make each other nervous. The hours went by when we were supposed to have gotten word that you were out of surgery. Nine-thirty went by, ten-thirty went by, eleven-thirty went by. We were starting to have fears that something had gone terribly wrong. Twelve-thirty went by. We didn't want to call Tim at first because we worried that the hospital might try and reach him at the same time. When we did finally call him, he had no news. We drove over to your apartment to wait with Tim for the call.

"A resident finally called Tim around one P.M. and just said 'Everything's fine. It's just going slowly.' I thought it was an out-and-out lie. Surgery wouldn't take three times longer than expected if everything was fine. As the surgery went on and on, it became increasingly obvious to Mom and me that there'd been an absolute disaster. They should have said something more on the phone, explained the truth. More hours passed around the kitchen table, talking in anxious generalities, worrying What if the surgeon's knife slipped?

"At five o'clock they finally called and said they'd finished. They said they thought they'd gotten the tumor just as they were finishing. It sounded like complete bullshit. They had operated as long as they could and then they had stopped. It would be the greatest coincidence if they had found the tumor at the last minute." His eyes filled with tears. "They didn't know how serious it was. . . . Can we quit?" he asked, wanting to end the painful memories.

When I finally woke up and could see a corner of the white walls with a clock in the neurosurgical intensive care unit, it was 7:30 at night. I was unaware that the reason I could see so little was that my wrists and ankles were strapped to the bed — preventing me from moving — and a bandage covered one eye. I wondered if I had forgotten most of the day, if the preoperative and operative medications had given me amnesia as Bruce had warned they might.

Soon Dr. Barrows's face appeared in the small area I could see. As he approached, I asked, "How long was the surgery?"

"It took ten hours, Jody. You got up here about a half hour ago."

As soon as he said ten hours, I knew something had gone terribly wrong. I tried to focus on what had happened, but my mind came in and out of morphine-induced delirium. The morphine was only enough to take the edge off the pain from the surgery, which was immeasurably worse than any pain I had ever had. Through the pain I tried to see Dr. Barrows clearly.

As his face came back into focus, he was saying, "It took ten hours because we had trouble finding the hemangioma. At the end we took something out, but I don't think we got the hemangioma."

Well, what do you say? I was getting very little medication to control the pain, in part because after neurosurgery it is essential to observe a patient's mental functioning and that functioning can be clouded by painkillers, and probably also in part out of a misunderstanding of how morphine works. In the midst of what would be a night of torture, Dr. Barrows had decided to tell me that they could not find what they went after, that this simple hour-and-a-half surgery had somehow lasted ten hours and had not been so simple, and that maybe it was all for far worse than nothing. Was it bad timing for Dr. Barrows to break the news when he did? That is not actually what I thought at the time. The information registered, but without reaction or response. I was too busy fighting the battle at hand, fighting the second hand on the clock, with my teeth and hands clenched, waiting for the minutes to pass until I could have more pain medication. One fact stuck with me. In his remarks was buried the idea that they had taken out a piece of my healthy brain. After all, he said they had taken something out, and he did not think it was the vascular tumor. Then what the hell was it?

Some undetermined amount of time passed, and the nurse had slipped into the space that I could see.

"Your parents are here. Do you want visitors?"

"No, not yet," I said, shaking my head, fighting back the tears. I knew I had no resources left to be reassuring to anyone else, and I did not want them to see what state I was in. As I closed my eyes, hallucinations returned.

The pain was unbearable. I had no energy to cry, no energy to scream. My whole body was racked with the intensity of the pain. Pain thresholds are odd. Are some people's higher because they experience less pain or are better at handling the pain? I do not believe that a high threshold is a badge of honor. Nonetheless, I had always been told that I had a high one. But this pain was terrifying.

The doctors were limiting the morphine I could receive to every two hours, even though morphine has a half-life of less than an hour when given intravenously; that means more than half of the dose is gone from the blood in an hour. Immediately after the morphine, the pain would be dulled enough that I could drift into a half-awake state. In that state, I would close my eyes, and the hallucinations would return: haunting visual hallucinations, abstract Rorschach blots representing pure terror, ceaselessly coming back in waves. Most horrifying of all was the fact that there was nowhere to run. Each time that the morphine dulled the pain enough to close my eyes, the hallucinations were there, waiting to sabotage any moment of peace. Had I gone insane?

As the minutes passed, the morphine would wear off. An hour later it would have barely any effect left, and I would be jolted back into the full battle against pain. Since that time, public discussions of physician inadequacy of pain control have become more frequent. A *New York Times* article written by two physicians discussed how doctors misunderstand pain, have inadequate knowledge about treating pain, and do not use the understanding of pain control they do have. As a specific example, they cited the fact that morphine is commonly dosed too infrequently to be effective.

Strapped into the bed, there was nowhere to move. There were only two things within sight: the white ceiling and the clock. I would grasp the steel rail of the bed, squeeze as tightly as I could, and watch the second hand of the clock tick away the excruciating minutes until the nurse's face would pop in again.

Nothing can erase the horrors of that night from my mind. They wiped out most of my innocence about bravery.

"Is it time yet, is it time yet?"

"No, not yet."

"Is it time now?"

"No, not yet."

"How much longer?"

"An hour."

I do not know how much I was trying to be a "good patient," which is too often defined as a compliant one, and how much the fight for survival, the hallucinations, and the pain silenced me. In any event, I said little more.

Tim saw me during this time, my teeth clenched, my knuckles white from squeezing the handrails, and my eyes filled equally with tears and horror. He sized up the intensive care unit, a small room with old beds crowded next to each other, tiny windows, old equipment, and pale green paint commonly used in institutions four decades ago. He asked the nurses about getting me more pain medication. They replied simply, "We're sorry, but she's getting as much as has been ordered." He knew how the system worked. He knew that the nurses could call the resident if they chose and ask for more pain medication. Then it would be up to the resident. But his request for the possible was answered routinely, as though it were impossible.

I had finally fallen asleep when I was awakened for the next neurologic check.

"What date is today?"

"July seventh."

"What time of day is it?"

"Night."

"What is your name?"

"Jody Heymann."

"Where are you?"

Pausing between words, I replied, "University Hospital. Didn't I answer these questions before?"

"Yes, but we have to keep doing it every hour. Press down with your foot. Okay. Press down with the other foot."

"Can I have some pain medicine yet?" I quietly pleaded.

"No, not yet. Squeeze my right hand. Good job! Squeeze my left hand."

It was a relief to have at least a few minutes awake without hallucinations.

Moments later, a man whom I did not know came in. His scrubs and the stethoscope around his neck made him look like a surgical resident. He did not introduce himself, but he repeated the test.

"Push down on your right foot. Okay. Push down on your left foot. You did well in the surgery. We took several samples of brain tissue to see what they were."

That remark registered. What had they taken? If it wasn't the hemangioma, then what was it? Would I be different now? Why several samples? I wanted them back. The resident left.

It was back to the cycle of morphine, the ever present but temporarily dulled pain, the fatigue leading to closed eyes and hallucinations, then the pain, jolting me awake again. The night passed that way. I was uncertain which to dread more — the onset of the pain or the hallucinations. When a nurse appeared in the white corner of the ICU that I could see, we would have brief interchanges.

"Do you remember any of the surgery, Jody?"

"No, I really don't remember anything until I woke up here. Except for one part in the operating room, with me lying flat on the table, the surgeons walking around preparing, and the anesthesiologist at my wrist trying again and again to get the arterial line in. Then another doctor trying. I think they stuck me seven times. I don't know if it was a dream or if I really remember it, because I don't remember anything else."

The next day, I would learn the truth as I counted the scars on my wrist: one, two, three, four, five, six, yes, seven. Months later, when we put arterial lines into babies too young to talk, some physicians said it was not a painful procedure and recommended doing it without local anesthesia. Paul, a senior resident, knew better. Uncomplaining Paul took months to recover from a car accident in Brazil. He had not forgotten being a patient. He remembered the pain of doctors attempting to place an arterial line without local anesthesia. But most of the doctors working with us knew little about what patients experience on a day-to-day basis.

The second hand went slowly. Six hours had passed since I had first woken up. The nurse was back to ask, "What's your name? Do you know where we are?"

"Do you know how long the pain lasts like this?" I asked, thinking that if there was an end in sight, it would be easier to survive, even if it meant watching the second hand of the clock in the narrow view I continued to have through one unbandaged swollen eye.

"No, I am afraid I really don't have any idea."

She was afraid? Why don't they know? Doesn't anyone ever ask patients?

Grasping for any footing in the quicksand, I asked, "Well, do you think it will be better in two or three days?"

Silence.

The night went by far more slowly than the thirty hours of labor for my son's birth. But this was a different kind of waiting as well as a different kind of pain; it was like being stuck in a horror movie. As failed sleep made the fatigue deepen, it grew impossible to tell wakefulness from sleep, except for the dreams. I dreamed I was in a race, and the race started but I could not get anywhere. When I awoke still strapped to the bed, I remembered I really could not move.

The next day, my parents came again to the intensive care unit. Seeing that I looked as bad as the others in the intensive care unit depressed my parents. One eye was covered by the

large bandage encircling my head; the other was blackened and
swollen half shut. But worse than the discoloration and swelling was the vacancy they highlighted in my gaze. Worse than
the restraints strapping my limbs was their superfluousness; my
limbs were stiffened and immobilized from pain. My mother
was the first to notice that the unbandaged half of my face did
not move, but she remained silent about it.

On July 8, Dr. Barrows offered what he thought was a gift. "I
thought I'd discharge you from the ICU today. It's on the early
side, but you're a doctor. You know how the hospital is on the
weekend. If I don't discharge you today, you could be in here
two more days."

Every other time I had been sick and had been offered a
choice, I had fought to be discharged from the hospital as
soon as possible. I was raised to push myself hard. But,
despite having overstepped my limits at other times, this time
I knew that being let out early would be no gift. It was
obvious even to me.

The principal difference between a regular hospital room
and one in an intensive care unit is that nurses have less time to
provide care for patients in regular rooms because each nurse
has to care for many more patients. I was less self-sufficient
than a newborn. At least a newborn can urinate and swallow on
his own. I had a Foley catheter inserted into my bladder to
catch urine, required intravenous fluids because I could not
drink or eat on my own, was vomiting repeatedly, and had
balloons inflating and deflating regularly around my legs to
prevent blood clots because I could not move. The visual
hallucinations continued whenever I closed my eyes, stealing
away any rest and replacing it with dread.

If Dr. Barrows truly did face a dilemma about whether to
discharge me too early or too late from the intensive care unit

merely because it was the weekend, then it adds another to the list of indictments against hospitals for not being structured around patient care. Even the cheapest motel can manage to have people arrive and leave on the weekend.

I did not say anything about the move. Stoic or not, most patients would not respond. Too sick to articulate their feelings or concerns readily, patients are placed in a position of inequality where the highest compliment given them is not that they are thoughtful partners in care but rather compliant patients.

Haunted by the hallucinations, fearing they might be a permanent result of the surgery, I did ask despondently, "Dr. Barrows, how long will I have the hallucinations?"

"I don't know. I don't know anyone who has had them."

Had they ever asked patients about their experiences? I wondered again silently. In how many cases had he operated for ten hours on the temporal lobe?

"I do not have any idea what would cause them," Dr. Barrows continued.

I had some ideas. "They must be related to the surgery. I didn't have them before. Maybe they're from ten hours of manipulating the temporal lobe." He looked doubtful. "Or maybe the anesthesia." It was the look doctors so often give, that doubtful look when a patient experiences something that the doctor does not understand.

In some cultures, if an individual is sick with something you do not understand, then a witch caused the illness. In our medical culture, if doctors do not understand a symptom, the patient is crazy, or making the symptom up, "it's all in their head."

Months before, I had put more faith in doctors when they disregarded a physical foundation for symptoms than I do now. During the spring before my first seizure, I had allowed doctors to rapidly dismiss my concerns about headaches. At first I ignored the headaches too because I had heard over and over again, "Oh, you know medical students, whenever they get headaches, they think they have a brain tumor." As the headaches grew more frequent and harder to ignore, I called an internist. He took the second-most common medical approach to ignorance. Over the phone he diagnosed stress since I was writing both a master's and doctoral thesis. Sensing the headaches were more severe than stress-based headaches, but needing to place my trust in the physician caring for me, I traded trusting myself for trusting him. I was not yet aware of how often doctors push patients and their families into that unnecessary and catastrophic trade.

Now, I couldn't help but think that the hallucinations that continued every time I closed my eyes were somehow related to the surgery.

On July 10, three days after the surgery, Dr. Barrows sent me for a repeat MRI of my brain. Tim stood by my stretcher and held my hand in the empty hallway as he had for the previous MRI. After the technician took me inside, Tim sat in a booth where a screen flashes images of the inside of the brain as the computer generates them. The process is miraculous but time-consuming. A scan of the brain may take forty-five minutes.

Tim sat silently next to the radiologist watching the images come up on the screen. As the imager, taking imaginary slices or cuts of brain, came to my temporal lobe, discouragement swept over his face. Tim was not a radiologist, but it was plain to see: the abnormal area of tumor had not changed at all since before the surgery. The radiologist said he could not give an official reading until he went over the scan with his superior.

Later that day, Dr. Barrows came into my room without his usual entourage of five residents. He pulled up a chair next to the bed and moved his hand somewhat nervously.

"Jody, it appears from the new MRI, like I suspected, that we didn't get the hemangioma. We need to go back in for more surgery." He was an excellent physician used to doing an excellent job. He wanted to finish what he had started and set things right. He wanted to do it before I went home.

He explained that he now thought that the first MRI had been taken at slightly different angles at Regional Medical Center. Because of that, they had opened the skull in the wrong place. When they were operating, they had realized that the tumor was at the very edge of their surgical field, inaccessible under the flap of skull.

He explained that he would be away for a few days but could do it as soon as he got back. He knew where the hemangioma was. He was certain that he would get it this time.

The questions exploded silently but violently. Why hadn't they repeated Regional's MRI before the surgery if there can be variation in techniques between hospitals? Tim and I knew how common it was for surgeons to repeat radiologic exams that have been performed at other hospitals. We had explicitly asked Dr. Barrows if he wanted the test repeated. When he had said the technique was standard and he could be sure by reading the landmarks of the brain on the map the MRI provided, we had believed him. If they did not repeat the MRI, why didn't they spend more time reading it so they would know where they were operating? Once they realized that the tumor was at the edge of the surgical field, why didn't they make the opening area bigger so they could just get it? Having a little more hair shaved off was a lot better than going through surgery twice.

But the only words I spoke were "It's okay. We're all human and we all make mistakes." I could tell from the situation as well as from listening to him talk how badly he felt. "It's always hard to be the person who makes the mistake and the person on whom the mistake is made, but it's unavoidable that it happens sometimes." The words were true, spoken by a new physician, aware of her own ability to make mistakes. But they belied the feelings of the patient who was occupying the same body.

Dr. Barrows knew better. "I'm amazed you're not more angry about this."

"Are you sure you can get it next time?"

"We can use stereotactics under CAT scan guidance. We'll put a metal halo around your head, and then we'll use the CAT scan to direct metal probes toward the mass."

After letting his answers about finding the hemangioma sink in, I asked quietly, "Are the risks any different the second time around?"

"I think there is a little more concern about it being near the motor strip. It could affect the strength of your facial movements on the left side, but I don't think it will affect your arm or leg." I tried to believe that it would be vanity not to go ahead because of a risk to facial movements, but deep down I knew facial strength was crucial to communication; it affects our daily interactions profoundly. If it had made sense to have the surgery the first time and if, as he assured me, the risks were no greater the second time and he was sure they would be able to get the hemangioma out, then it was rational to go ahead the second time. I also wanted to finish what we had started, to make things right.

The rational voice within me said aloud, "That makes sense. Let's do it as soon as you get back." What I meant was "Let's get it over with."

Amid ongoing severe pain, terror of round-the-clock hallucinations fresh in my mind, still too weak to walk and still unable to think clearly for more than five or ten minutes at a time, I dreaded the second surgery more than I had ever dreaded anything in my life.

There was nothing that came close. When I had malaria weekly and biweekly overseas, with fevers up to 105 degrees, I sometimes was too weak to walk, and had to be handed bodily by colleagues through a window of a crowded public bus so that I could get to the hospitals, hospitals where a ward might have fifty patients and one nurse, and half the patients had no bed. When I worked in Central America, I stayed up all night in a war zone listening to gunfire and at times fearing for my life. But I had never before feared losing my mind and I had never understood the expression pain worse than death. I had always hungered for life too much.

I still hungered for as full a life as possible and was ready to do whatever it took to lead that life. If having surgery again meant a fuller life, a better chance at contributing through my work, at working overseas again, at becoming pregnant without endangering the fetus, then I was ready to have it. But not with the same courage, brought on by the denial of vulnerability, with which I had faced the first operation. I wanted to get the surgery over with so that I could go on with life as soon as possible, so that the next weeks would not be overshadowed by dread of what lay ahead, so that I would not have to spend months recovering from the first operation only to have surgery again. I did not want to spend twice as long recovering, twice as long not being able to mother as I had before, twice as long having to ask Tim to carry a double load, twice as long not being able to work.

Tim was ready for us to go ahead with the second operation, too. My father's fears were exceeded only by his anger. He kept thinking, How dare this man. He has a life in his hands, and he's treating it with the gravity of a double-or-nothing crap shoot. The image my father could not shake was one that transcended more than two decades. My grandmother, to whom I had always been compared in values and temperament, had died suddenly, while still young, after two unnecessary operations followed each other in quick succession. The family diagnosis was that it had been too much for her.

Dr. Barrows continued to be exceptionally patient, good at listening and at answering questions. Visiting me in the hospital room, he would always say, "I know you'll have many questions every day. You may want to discuss the same ones again soon that we discussed today. Don't worry, I'll be back. If you want to ask the same questions, that's fine." He would continue, surrounded by residents, "It must be hard to remember many of the conversations we had right after the surgery. It's also hard to talk when seven people come into your room rounding. We'll have more time alone."

Four days after the first operation, I finally could tell the difference between day and night. "Tim, who has visited? Who has come and gone while I didn't know what was going on? I want to try and remember, so that I can thank them." The room was filled with bouquets; it smelled like a flower shop, but looked like a funeral home. I wanted to thank the many people who were giving me support but I didn't know how to begin. Conversations were difficult; my concentration lasted only minutes. And writing was next to impossible.

JULY 11, A.M.

(written in scrawl, barely legible now) I won't write long now because of the mental exhaustion, but I want to try and remember the truth of what this is like and not haze it over with the fog of time. It takes all my energy to concentrate and have a ten-minute conversation; even more to write one extremely loose, poorly worded set of reminders for the future like this. As hard as I try, I cannot read more than two pages of a novel at a time. The problem is fatigability, not dullness. I start clear and sharp but then fatigue within minutes to a state far beyond that I have ever arrived at by working 60 hour shifts in the hospital without sleep. . . . Mom just came, time for a visit with her. Dad says she is really worried. Hope I can calm her.

JULY 11, P.M.

(written on borrowed hospital paper) I cannot help but listen and look around this floor and feel extremely lucky. Lucky not to have one of the many grave diseases with high mortality and severe long-term deficits that people here are facing. Lucky not to have to face it alone. Visitors vanquish the dread.

LATER

Talked with Sarah, who is getting married soon, on the phone. Sarah said her mother wanted me to know she is praying for me. Sarah has been calling Tim for updates and relaying them to other friends. Mary calls Sarah from Europe for news, Todd from North Carolina. Many more flowers arrived with well-wishes. Tim and my parents told me of all the calls from family and friends they get each evening.

JULY 12, 4:30 A.M.

In the dream, the computer printer was not turned on as I ran toward it shouting for a friend not to take out the paper, which I had been working on. She took it out and threw it away. As I started running toward her and the paper in the terminal, they kept getting farther away. There was an escalator but there was dirt next to it, which I kept sliding down. As the route down to the printer and paper got longer, people started telling me to jump. As I took off in the air, the distance I had to jump became longer and longer. No one had expected the ground would fall away from under me.

It does not take a Jungian to understand this dream.

JULY 12, 10 P.M.

Vomiting, unable to keep down Decadron [the medication that decreases brain swelling].

JULY 12, MIDNIGHT

More vomiting. I am sure it is getting worse. Once you cannot keep down the Decadron, it is a vicious cycle. The brain swelling increases, and the vomiting from increased intra-cranial pressure goes up.

JULY 13, 2 A.M.

Vomiting every half hour now, unable to keep the Decadron down.

Janet, a nurse on the night shift, brought the medicine.

"Can I get the Decadron intravenously? That's how they were giving it to me up till six P.M. tonight. I have not kept any down for the last two doses."

When a patient "does not tolerate" oral medications, the medical euphemism for vomiting, changing back to intravenous doses is routine.

"Let me just check with the resident on call."

"Okay. Can . . . can I have the puke bucket again?" More vomiting. The room was dimly lit by the hallway light. As the emesis basin filled, I pushed the nurse call button above the bed. The nurses did not want me to walk the six feet to the bathroom entrance alone.

"What did he say?" I asked Janet, referring to the medicine, knowing that I would only be getting worse unless I had some Decadron.

"He wants to wait until morning rounds before he makes any changes."

Janet cared tenderly for me through the night as the vomiting increased to every fifteen minutes. Anyone who has been in the hospital knows that those who care for patients day in and day out are the nurses.

By five in the morning, I was vomiting up a brilliant green fluid that looked like antifreeze. It was bilious vomiting, caused by the gallbladder releasing bile into the small intestine. In severe vomiting, bile is what comes up after everything in the stomach has been vomited up.

With the training of a doctor and the vulnerability of a patient, I knew that the increasing headaches and bilious vomiting were clear signs of increased pressure inside the skull and that the most likely cause was postoperative brain swelling, which had been previously controlled by the Decadron. I also knew that signs of brain swelling are dangerous to ignore.

"Can you talk to the resident again? . . . Can you ask him . . . to come see me . . . please?" I gasped out in between vomiting. Hesitant as many patients are to press unwilling caretakers for help, I nonetheless thought if I could talk to the resident, if he would see how sick I was, maybe I could convince him.

She came back minutes later. "He is in the call room." I knew what that meant: he did not want to get out of bed. I did not care. A patient was really sick, and that is why doctors are in the hospital overnight.

"Janet, can . . . you please wake him up? . . . You can tell him . . . I asked you to." I got out only broken fragments as the retching was no longer intermittent.

He wandered into the semilit room in his blue scrubs, drowsily. "I really don't think that the Decadron has anything to do with your vomiting," he said, "but we will discuss it on rounds." He was not concerned enough to think about or offer an alternative explanation. He may have been too tired to do the right thing.

The next morning began with me sitting upright drooling vomit over my Johnny, an emesis basin constantly in hand. The day shift was on, and the nurse came two more times with medicine that I could never keep down. There was no chance of it when I could not even swallow my own saliva without vomiting. My head was pounding as the brain swelling increased unchecked, and my brain pressed hard against the skull.

At eleven, thirteen hours after the vomiting started, I called Tim. I had exhausted almost all other avenues, except calling an ambulance. I thought of a story I had been told about a man who went to the emergency room of a New York City hospital. He waited for hours while he was having a heart attack, unable to receive attention. Finally, he called an ambulance to take him to another hospital. When the ambulance driver arrived to pick the man up, he was stunned to find himself in a hospital emergency room. The ambulance driver brought the man's situation to the attention of the hospital staff, and the man finally received care. When I first heard the story, it had seemed sad, funny, and more than a little apocryphal. Now it seemed entirely credible and as ingenious as it was desperate.

"Tim, . . . I'm just puking all the time. . . . It's bilious vomit. . . . I know what's wrong. . . . I know it has to be increased intracranial pressure . . . but I can't get the resident to do anything about it. . . . I haven't been able to keep Decadron down," I explained, interrupting sentences with vomiting, working as a physician to describe the patient who was still untreated. "Tim, . . . can you call someone? . . . I am just too sick at this point . . . to do anything more. . . . I've really tried here."

With Tim's intervention, the attending physician covering for Dr. Barrows while he was out of town came in. As soon as he saw me and the constant fluorescent green vomiting, he ordered an emergency CAT scan of the brain. He began the intravenous Decadron immediately. Back on the stretcher, I was sent on another tour of the hospital ceilings that were so familiar now. As the technician and resident lifted me off the stretcher and onto the CAT scan, I was still vomiting persistently into one green kidney-shaped emesis basin after another.

Into the small area that I could see at the top of the walls, came, to my surprise, two familiar faces: Dr. Johnson and Dr. Feder, the physicians in charge of the medical student rotation and the residency at Children's Hospital, where I was scheduled to have begun work already, had come to visit. I waved as the conveyor belt electronically moved me into the doughnut hole of the CAT scan. I was lucky: I got to soak up the warmth of their brief visit, but they left looking sobered having seen the changes that had taken place.

With that episode of aseptic meningitis, Tim's and my attitude toward immediate further surgery began to shift. Finally, I understood that willpower alone was not enough to make me physically ready within days for more major surgery. Tim talked to his father, a cardiologist, who encouraged him to "let the dust settle before making a decision."

As the days passed, I gradually gained enough strength to walk alone to the bathroom six feet away and, after resting, to walk back to my bed. One morning as I stood up to walk, Richard, a fourth-year medical student, came into the room for his daily visit. He was dressed in a short white coat that distinguishes medical students and residents from attendings. He had used a patient ID band to place his name on the stethoscope he wore around his neck. Like kids wearing combat fatigues, many medical students use patient IDs to label their medical equipment; for them the IDs have no feelings of pain attached. Kind and thorough on each of his visits, he had come to do a complete physical exam. He listened with his stethoscope to my chest, then heart, and examined my abdomen as well as doing a full neurologic exam. He was the only physician or physician-in-training during my entire hospital stay who listened to my lungs and heart after the surgery. No one else bothered.

No one else asked about the things that mattered. The pain, the hallucinations, and the vomiting were all topics they avoided. Richard asked, "What happened to the picture of your son?" Spending extra time with each patient, he remembered details from their rooms. He had noticed the hard to miss eight-by-ten-inch picture of Ben on the wall. He had also immediately noticed and asked about its absence.

"The picture," I explained, "was on the wall because I was always thinking of him. That way I could see him and touch him and kiss him. The more days I've spent in the hospital, the harder it's been to be away from him, and I just couldn't take his picture up on the wall anymore. . . . Seeing him in his picture and not being able to see him in person."

"The separation has been really hard?"

"Yeah, . . . he's less than one year old and we were just with each other all the time. When he needed something, he was there screaming 'Mommy, Mommy, Ma, Ma, Ma, Ma.' It's hard not to be there to respond. It's even harder to think about going home not physically strong enough yet to be able to pick him up when all he will want is to be picked up and held. The one thing I have been told is to limit my bending over and picking up any weight. I did that a hundred times a day — to pick up a bundle of hugs."

Richard finished his exam quietly.

The messages about what had been removed from my brain were conflicting. Dr. Barrows stuck to the story that only one small piece of tissue had been removed. But nagging away at me was the recollection of the resident's report in the intensive care unit that several pieces of brain tissue had been removed. Like other patients who have gone through surgery or who have had a disease that has caused them to lose something, I worried about whether I would be the same person as before or somehow less.

Reassurances and even respectful remarks always seemed to be a double-edged sword. A friend passed on what Susan, impressed with how I had managed medical school, motherhood, and graduate school, had said: "Of all the brains, why did this have to happen to hers?" The story was told as a compliment, but it contained a clear conception people have of brain surgery: the person will never be the same.

My aunt and uncle came to visit. They asked about the prospects of new surgery. I told them all the pros and cons in as much medical and analytical detail as I could. At the end, my uncle said, "I am amazed at your comprehension of the complexities." It is always hard to know what to make of someone's amazement that you can think.

Dr. Barrows's attitude about surgery shifted when the first pathologic report came back. The report stated that the tissue he removed was benign, a cavernous hemangioma. His desire to reoperate had been based on his belief that he had not removed any of the hemangioma and in the importance of making a pathologic diagnosis to ensure that the tumor was not cancerous. Happily surprised by the fact that the report seemed to provide a diagnosis, he was ready to send me home.

JULY 15

I'm very excited about the prospect of going home tomorrow. I can't wait to see Benjamin and try to get on my feet. Tim and my parents claim I started the rumor that I was getting discharged tomorrow just so I could get myself out.

With the help of a nurse, I walked all the way down the hall to the shower, where she had placed a seat by the handrails for me. She washed my hair, still matted with blood and colored by vomit, with perfumed shampoo.

After taking a seated shower and being assisted back to my room, I looked in the mirror for the first time at a head without bandages and hair clean of blood. The smile in the mirror turned uncontrollably into a grimace as I noticed how contorted it was. Only half of my facial muscles were moving as they once had. The right cheek sagged and the right side of my lips drooped, but they did move. Most noticeable of all was that for the first time in several years, my right forehead was free of wrinkles. It was also free of movement.

I recalled my surgery rotation in medical school. Lesson number one: when operating on the face, be careful not to destroy the facial nerve since that will give the patient a palsy. Facial palsies paralyze that crucial foundation of communication — the ability to smile, to frown, to express compassion or complacency without saying a word.

Bruce, the physician's assistant who had prepared me for surgery, came in to prepare me for discharge. "So, are you happy about going home?"

"I can't wait. You know that. I've been dying to get home, but I just noticed this about my face," I said, pointing. "My facial nerve isn't working. Did it get cut in the surgery?"

"Let me look," Bruce replied. "Nobody has mentioned anything about it. Lift up your eyebrows. You're right. It could be cut, but it also could be the result of being stretched for ten hours. We won't know for a couple of months."

"Why didn't anyone notice it? Why did I have to discover it myself in the bathroom?" Some of the anger at everything that had gone wrong sneaked past the guards that usually held such comments at bay.

"Well, maybe they didn't notice," Bruce suggested.

"Maybe they didn't notice" is a phrase that is joked about in medical school. When people write WNL after a physical exam, it is supposed to mean "within normal limits," but it also means "we never looked." Had no one checked for something so basic? Or had they noticed and said nothing about it?

The medical chart discharge summary, on July 16, began "The patient is a 25-year-old right-handed woman with no past significant medical history who presented with a generalized seizure on 6/16/89, after several months of headache . . ."

I was a twenty-nine-year-old woman. Details.

The discharge summary continued: "Post-operative MRI showed the lesion is still present in the right temporal lobe. This was discussed with the patient and plans were made approximately one and a half weeks later to have the patient return for re-operation with stereotactic guidance. There were no complications."

No complications? It was either a matter of trying to protect themselves or of opinion. What did they think about surgery that lasted an additional eight hours (six times as long as expected), aseptic meningitis, a facial nerve palsy, and the failure to remove all of the hemangioma they went in to get?

CHAPTER FOUR

The Struggle to Stand

I have had dreams, and I have had
nightmares. I overcame the nightmares
because of the dreams.

—*Jonas Salk, M.D.*

O<small>N JULY</small> 16, the day of my discharge, I woke up early and got dressed as fast as I could. I sat in the small six-by-eight-foot hospital room waiting anxiously to be discharged, staring at the walls now blank again; the get well cards had been taken down. Somehow, even after all those months of working in hospitals, I had no idea how long it takes to get discharged. The hours crept by like tortoises in a slow race: six . . . seven . . . eight . . . nine . . . ten . . . eleven o'clock. Still nothing. I thought all they had to do was sign a sheet that said "Discharge." Twelve . . . one o'clock. The day that was so important to me — to be well enough to go back home to see Ben, to go running from hell — was just an ordinary day for everyone working in the hospital. My discharge was not high on their list; I understood that. But it seemed so simple: just a few signatures. Seven hours after getting up, I asked the day nurse a second time when I would be able to go.

"We are waiting for the residents to write the prescriptions."

"If they just tell me what I need to take, I can get them written," I volunteered.

"No. They can't do that. They'll get to it when they have time." Prescriptions take only a few minutes to write.

The delay was so hard to understand as a patient. The doctors had said I could leave first thing in the morning. It's surprising how much it hurts once one's expectations are set. I was desperate to leave, desperate to see my son.

Yet the fault did not lie with the residents, who are so busy that they eat lunch in the elevator and urinate in a bathroom en route to the next patient. The problem lies in a system that pits the basic needs of residents against the simple hopes of patients, a system that treats the passing of time as imperceptible to patients and their families, a system that often saves money by cutting human resources regardless of cost and keeps technology regardless of benefits.

My father had come to the hospital to help Tim pack up the contents of my room. When Tim had taken me to the hospital, I had had just the clothes on my back and a medical insurance card, which was the key to admission. Leaving, we looked like a flower shop ready to set up on the street.

When the prescriptions were at last signed eight hours later, my adrenaline was so high that I would not wait for a wheelchair, after being told it would take another hour for one to arrive. Foolhardy and ambitious, having walked fifty feet up and down the corridor, I was convinced I could walk to the car. No wonder many hospitals have rules that patients have to be taken to the door in a wheelchair. It was the first, but not the last, time I would overestimate my strength. Pregnant women often try to squeeze through a space that they once would have fit through but that is now far too small. Just as their minds are slow to adjust to the growth of pregnancy, my mind was slow to understand fully the physical limitations that followed surgery.

We walked a hundred yards until I was about to faint. I sat down for a brief moment, and then was back up again, walking for home like it was a run for life. Another hundred yards and back sitting down again. It would either be a voluntary sit or an involuntary fall after losing consciousness. Another hundred yards, another stop. Another hundred yards, stop, sit, sinking to the realization that when patients are discharged it does not mean they are well. Finally, the car. The station wagon was equipped with front seats that can be placed in a near horizontal position. I lay down on the seat and anticipated seeing Ben. For the first time since leaving the hospital bed, my head stopped spinning.

Ben was emotional at reunions. Earlier that spring, when Tim and I returned from our first overnight absence to retrieve Ben from his adoring grandparents, Ben puffed up his plump cheeks and sat with his bottom lip rapidly quivering. He waited for us to lift him up and hold him, the three of us entangled in an embrace, before screaming and smiling at the same time.

The difference this time was that I could neither pick him up nor stand up and hold him. He was frightened and confused. A different mother had come back, her head partially shaven and scarred, her face half paralyzed, her skin hanging loosely from atrophied arms and legs. His initial "Ma, Ma, Ma, Ma," the closest he could come with a one-year-old's vocabulary to demanding to be picked up, was rapidly replaced by soft, sad cries as he realized the incomprehensible, that I could not — would not, in his eyes — pick him up or hold his strong, squirming body while standing.

I felt like the child who blows bubbles, and every bubble she blows a bully runs up to burst. My first dream had been to graduate from medical school and start an internship in pediatrics. My second one, after the seizure and discovery of the hemangioma, had been to undergo a single operation that would lead to a surgical cure. The last dream had been to go home strong enough to care for myself and my son.

Concerns for Ben that had sprouted in the hospital grew rapidly. His first birthday was only a few days away. I became increasingly worried about how to throw him a birthday party that would make him happy. Now, it is easy to say that the worries were wildly irrational: How, for example, would a one-year-old even know if we celebrated his birthday on time? But I latched on to the idea, and kept worrying that my ill health might affect his happiness, or that the abnormality of my life might affect the normality of his.

More surprising than either Ben's or my response was my lack of preparation. In *Living with Chronic Illness,* the author devotes a whole chapter to the impact of illness on parenting (Register 1987). Parents speak of the "very traumatic" experience when "here you are, this new mother and you can't even hold your baby," or when they "can't even spend a day at the circus" with an older child. Yet, as common and essential as these experiences are, they were neither in my medical school curriculum nor raised with me as a patient.

That night, I recognized the amount of noise in the hospital when it was replaced by near silence at home. Just before leaving the hospital, the staples in the surgical incision were removed. At home, I was able at last to try lying on my right side when a grinding clicking aroused me. Click . . . click . . . click . . . click . . . click. Slowly at first, and then in rapid succession. During the surgery, a portion of my skull had been replaced with an artificial plate. The grinding was the sound of the plate pressing inward against the skull. As I rolled off my right side, it would grind back in reverse. Click . . . click . . . click . . . click . . . click, as my brain, pressure relieved, pushed the plate back into its original position. Falling back asleep, I would unconsciously roll onto my right side again until I was woken by the rapid-fire clicks starting again like a fan off balance.

Each morning started with a few cherished moments with Ben as soon as he awoke. During the first few days home, I would expend all my energy in those first few minutes of the day. Then the fatigue rolled in as unstoppable as fog, exacting a high price for those few moments of mental clarity and physical exuberance, including the little time holding Ben. Afterward, while I lay there doing nothing, hours passed that on a healthy day would have driven me crazy. But now, doing nothing took so much energy that it seemed like an activity. At the end of a morning of doing nothing but thinking — no reading, no radio, no television, no visitors — the exhaustion felt like the end of a marathon I had failed to train for.

The seizure, the surgery, and the hospital stay had been unable to penetrate the denial of vulnerability built during medical training as piercingly as those first days at home. We lived in a small apartment: a double bed filled three-quarters of the master bedroom, Ben's bedroom door was across a two-foot hallway from ours, and the living room and bathroom were both three feet away from our bedroom. Yet compared to a hospital room, the apartment was as large and unmanageable as the White House would have been. I was too weak to bring Ben from his room to mine, too weak to walk to the bathroom without sitting down en route, and too weak to reach the kitchen for water without making many stops.

The first postoperative days at home are not covered in any medical school curriculum. At medical school, we do not discuss whether patients will be able to make it to the bathroom alone, to the kitchen to get water, to the phone to get help, and, if not, who will help them. We do not discuss what to do if patients are single or if they are raising children or caring for the elderly. We do not discuss who will take care of someone when physicians discharge their duties along with their patient from the hospital.

As residents, we are too busy. We rarely think of discussing this adjustment with patients, let alone helping with it, unless the patients have been dependent on others before they came to the hospital: a young child, an elderly person living in a nursing home, an institutionalized adult where the institution demands a report before it will accept the patient back. We forget the large number of people whom we take in who live independently when they enter, but after we are done with them — with our surgery, with our multiple medications, with our cures — leave unable to live independently, at least for a time.

My family took care of me those first few weeks, a fact for which I will be forever grateful. Roles were reversed. When my brother and I were growing up, my mother was at home, went to school, and did volunteer work. We followed my father as he transferred from one job to the next in the U.S. government and in academia. While committed to his work, he let his children know that whenever we needed him, he would drop everything he was doing and be with us. He was a tremendous source of stability and love in our lives. Yet he spent the majority of his time at work. The daily nurturing, the wiping of crayons off the walls and tears off our faces, came from my mother. Jell-O and toast on a tray in bed on a sick day home from school was her specialty.

When we graduated from high school, my mother went back to work full-time. Now, earlier in her career than my father, she had less flexibility. Now, she stayed at work. My father, an academic who could read and write anywhere, took his turn at making tea and toast, bringing the comforts of deep love, and watching on helplessly as a child was sick.

My cousin Danny also came to help. Danny, born on my twelfth birthday, was the first cousin for whom I can remember babysitting. I remember lying down on the living room floor as my aunt and uncle finished getting dressed to go out to dinner. Danny crawled up my legs, onto my chest, and grabbed me with one groping hand.

"What's this?" he asked, naturally uninhibited and inquisitive.

My uncle, a psychiatrist, made mute by the question and my own early adolescence, gasped as he fixed his cuff links.

"It's a breast," I replied without hesitation, more surprised by the adult's awkwardness than the toddler's innocence.

Now a college student, Danny spent the next several weeks taking care of multiply handicapped blind children in the morning and me in the afternoon. The tables had turned. The boy was a man, and I was sicker than I had imagined possible. Somehow when you have always been able to bounce back fast, when you have been able to work through serious illnesses before, it is as hard to imagine yourself disabled until you are as it is to imagine yourself dead. The intellectual exercise is possible, but it is no more than that. The exercise does not get through the concrete fortifications of denial.

Medical training had only added confidence to my ignorance of recovery. As physicians in training, we thought we knew what it was about. After all, we saw post-op patients all the time. Somehow, it never occurred to us that what we saw in the hospital and in rare twenty-minute outpatient visits did not resemble at all what went on for patients at home.

Exhaustion, pain, and mental fatigue limit written words and reading for now to short spurts of saved-up energy. So many thoughts. So many thanks for such incredibly loving family and friends.

That is all that I wrote for days. My father had given me books on tape to listen to during the day, but, fatigued past concentration, I could not follow even the simplest story. Nor was visiting with friends possible if visiting was used in the usual sense of a two-way conversation. Lying in the comforting presence of quiet friendship was closer to my abilities. For the only time in my life, just lying in bed was enough to keep me busy all day without boredom. Awake, asleep, awake, asleep, an unending pattern repeated a half dozen times throughout the day.

At first, I fought the fatigue every waking moment. I had been taught to deny illness and fatigue. Other physicians have described the lessons of a medical education this way: "We work all night; we're taught we can push our bodies to do anything. It's hard to understand when patients can't make themselves get on with their life." I was not so explicitly aware of the effect of training on me, but I had heard the same message of invulnerability — a remarkable message considering physicians deal daily with life-changing illnesses. How illness, chronic conditions, or disability changed people's daily lives had not been part of my medical education. But it was now.

Within a few days of getting out of the hospital, the weddings of two close friends, Sarah and Charlotte, were scheduled. Tim and I argued back and forth about the first wedding.

"Sarah and John will understand. They are not expecting you to be there. You do not have to go, Jody," Tim said in an exasperated voice.

"I know, Tim. I know they would understand, but I keep thinking about how weddings are once in a lifetime events, and you always have special memories of sharing them with your close friends. I really want to be able to go and share this time with them."

"But Jody, you can barely sit up for fifteen minutes. How

do you expect to make it through a wedding?" he asked, thinking logic would work.

"I can lie down during the drive there, and Sarah's mother offered to let me lie in the house until the wedding starts. Then I'll just go to the wedding. If worse comes to worst, at least I can sit through the wedding. That'll be only fifteen minutes."

As a child in the fourth grade attending parochial school, I was given a pendant with a mustard seed in it and a reminder that if you have enough faith to fill a mustard seed, you can move mountains. I believed that and still do, if you're given enough time.

I had tried to figure out before the wedding whether the telephoned offer of a place to rest had been out of Sarah's mother's earnest desire for me to come or out of accommodation, whether my efforts to attend the wedding would be welcomed or an unintended imposition. I went hoping that my coming would let Sarah, John, and their families know how much I cared.

The first shock came ten minutes into the car ride. I could not sit up any longer. So I lowered the seat into the horizontal position. Every time we struck a pothole in the road, a sharp pain shot through the right side of my head. Coming back out of the pothole, the clicking of the plate adjusting its position started: click . . . click . . . click . . . click . . . click . . . click . . . click, as I imagined it pushing in and out from my brain like two seven-year-old boys fighting for space in the backseat of the car. An hour and a half later, exhausted from the pain and cacophony inside my head, we arrived at Falmouth.

At the time, it surprised me that with everything else she was doing that afternoon — welcoming family and friends, getting ready for the wedding on the grassy point overlooking the ocean — Sarah's mother immediately offered me a place to lie down. It never occurred to me until I saw pictures of the wedding what I must have looked like when I arrived. The picture showed it clearly: a thin woman who had lost twenty pounds in a month, her skin hanging loosely from her arms and legs where the muscles had atrophied, her head shaved on the right, with a long scar burning red from the recently removed staples.

Into the upstairs bedroom with the sloping ceilings of a small Cape Cod summer house friends kept walking, bending over not to bump their heads, to say hello. Those moments were joyous, joyous to share life, to see friends, to have minutes of pure happiness after such pure hell. It took me ten minutes to walk the hundred yards to the green outcropping over the ocean, where the wedding took place. In the bright sunlight, sharp pain returned, a marked reminder of the photophobia that results from irritation of the brain's meningeal covering. I had not been outside for two weeks. No one had spoken the simple words of caution before I left the hospital: you will not want to eat; you will not be able to sleep; the sun will shoot pains through your eyes; you will not be able to open your jaw more than half an inch because of the injury to the muscles. Had the physicians listened enough to patients to know what to expect? Tim got his sunglasses out of the car and I wore them, feeling conspicuous but relieved as the pain subsided.

For the three days following Sarah's wedding, I had deep setbacks in store. I had tried to cheat the God of recovery and the pace he set. Now he would make me pay. Unable to get out of bed the first day, the second day barely sitting for minutes at a time. Then the third day, as signs of life were beginning to return, it was time for a debate about the second wedding. Before the surgery, Charlotte had planned for me to be one of her bridesmaids.

"Charlotte's wedding is tomorrow. I told her I probably could not be part of the wedding party, but that we could still go."

Tim started with reasoning, recognizing that I was a slow learner. "Jody, Charlotte will understand if you don't go," he said, repeating the words that he had used with Sarah's wedding. "You saw what happened with Sarah's wedding. You were there for a few hours and then paid for it for days." He was sitting at the foot of the bed where I was lying, still working on recovering strength from the last escapade.

"I know, Tim, but it was worth it," I said, laughing at my own insanity. "Besides, seriously," I said, as if by saying "seriously" he would take me seriously, "I was going to be a bridesmaid. The least I can do is go and be part of the wedding that she asked me to be in." The debate went on, and it made me, if nothing else, relinquish any remaining thoughts of trying still to be a bridesmaid. At least I recognized that it would not be a great wedding present for Charlotte to have someone in her bridal party pass out at her side.

On Sunday, we went off to the suburb where Charlotte's father-in-law lived. I went up to the second floor of the colonial house and stood behind Charlotte quietly. Seeing a shadow in the mirror, she turned around in her wedding gown while pinning her hair and saw me. She squealed, "Oh, you came," with such delight that it made it all worthwhile.

The wedding was on a well-manicured lawn behind the house. Since I'd been feeling dizzy before the wedding, Tim and I sat in the back row so as to be unobtrusive if we needed to leave. Pleased to have been able to participate in the wedding, even from a distance, and knowing it wouldn't be possible to push much further, Tim and I drove home soon afterward.

JULY 25

These are very discouraging days.

Haven't been able to sleep. Can't think or communicate readily, only slowly and with great effort. Frustrated at not being able to do anything all day, scared, anxious, not knowing how long this degree of disability will last: a day, a week, longer, a lifetime. Wishing I knew what caused it so I would know if it was serious. It has come on so abruptly. At the weddings I seemed to be doing so well.

It took four hours to write those words.

My mother was frightened by my inability to find common words. It was visible as well as audible. She would watch me pause and close my eyes to search for a word. Even in the morning, her conversations with me progressed haltingly as every second or third sentence was interrupted by a search.

After I had left the hospital, Tim and I could no longer avoid misunderstandings. The power of the misunderstandings came from their origin in love and need. In the evenings, fatigued, I was often pessimistic when Tim arrived home from work. I needed help for everything, yet I did not know how to ask for it, and was afraid of not knowing how long Tim would love me as a partner, dependent for every activity of daily living. The fear was made desperate by the dual uncertainties of knowing neither how long I would be disabled nor what I could give in return.

Tim loved me and did not want to see me sick. He shielded himself with a strong defense of denial. In medical school, when autonomic Guillain-Barré syndrome suddenly made it impossible for me to sit or stand, I was hospitalized where Tim worked. Full days would go by without my hearing from him; I would call at nine at night only to hear him explain he had been too busy to visit me. He had been busy and he had made himself more so, not wanting to see me too sick. With the seizure and surgery, he came through for every crisis, but as soon as possible, he relinquished any caretaking role and retreated to the safe hideaway of his work, as many husbands in similar circumstances had before him and many more wives might have done, had it been socially acceptable for them to do so.

Silent denial seduced both Tim and me at first until it became increasingly threatening. I facilitated his denial with my own efforts to keep silent at first about each new set of difficulties and to stubbornly seek to attempt the nearly impossible alone. It was only after running full speed into brick walls that I called for help.

Gradually we managed to break the silence. The process was nothing more mysterious than talking to each other about what we each feared, needed, and could do. The healing of communication was no more rapid and no less vital than the rest of recovery. Forced to develop ever deeper levels of frank communication, fueled by the profound trust that results from surviving experiences that are threatening to oneself and threatening to a partnership, our relationship became permanently stronger.

I was still not strong enough to write more than phrases, but I wanted to write them down as reminders:

Notes for when I am taking care of patients:
There are times when you are so sick . . . with delirium, the isolation from time and person caused by uncontrolled pain . . . that what you say no longer comes from who you are. It does not reflect your beliefs, feelings, your soul. It is a symptom of the state you are in.

It is particularly hard dealing with the indefiniteness . . . Will I need more surgery? . . . More treatment? . . . How much will my health improve? . . . How long before I can return to a normal life, if ever? . . . Will it be a normal life like before, forever, or only for a period? How hard it must be for patients with life-threatening diseases.

As the discharge summary so clearly stated, the doctors sent me home fully expecting that I would come back for a second operation. This time, my whole family was a little more leery. My grandfather repeated what had been one of his dictums for decades: "Fool me once, shame on you; fool me twice, shame on me." None of us could face my going back only to have the surgeons miss again.

Tim and I called Dr. Manson for another opinion. Should we worry? Was the fact that the surgeons missed the tumor the first time so unreasonable that we should not go back to the same group? What did he think?

There are, in general, two approaches doctors take to this type of question. There are doctors who will never comment on another physician's work to the physician's patients. Then there are doctors who give their honest opinion to patients because they recognize it is important to the patients' future care for them to know the truth. We realized that only a minority of physicians would break the unspoken but binding vows of loyalty to other physicians in order to counsel a patient openly, but we hoped that we would be able to learn the truth as members of the brethren ourselves.

Dr. Manson clearly felt committed to silence. He recited the usual requiem: "I was not there, so I really cannot say," even though he had seen the films and consulted on the surgery previously. But concerned and compassionate, he offered to see us, to review the CAT scans and MRIs, and discuss the question of whether further surgery was indicated.

We went back to one of the older buildings of the hospital, where his office, with its wood and leather furniture, was located. As he looked at the MRIs, he said, "I'm not sure you have any hemangioma left."

Shocked, I asked stupidly, "Are you serious?" Tim just stared at him in disbelief. The implications were impossible to accept at first. Dr. Barrows had operated. He had come to the intensive care unit to say that he had missed the tumor after an operation six times its expected length. Consequently, he had planned a second operation. The operation was delayed in large part because of aseptic meningitis. Had it not been for that complication, he probably would have operated a second time to remove something that was no longer there.

"It's just too early to tell," Dr. Manson elaborated. "At this stage, what you see on the MRI could be either postsurgical changes or the hemangioma."

This was not the wonderful news that the miraculous disappearance of the hemangioma would have been. It was merely a warning. There was no way to know what was there and what was not there right now, not for a while at least.

Pausing frequently between words, dumbfounded I asked, "How long will it take before you can tell the difference between surgical scarring and the hemangioma?"

"Probably a couple of months. But you should be followed regularly over the next two to three months anyway because of the ring-enhancing lesion," he advised, referring to a circle on the CAT scan that could indicate a serious infection. He added cautiously, once more trying to avoid any conflicts with other physicians, "What did they tell you that was?"

"They thought it was probably a postoperative glial response, since I was not as sick as they thought I'd be if it had been an abscess." I repeated their response to what was a disturbing abnormality on the brain scan. The new abnormality clearly was related to the surgery. Whether or not there was an infection they did not know. They just worried and waited.

Tim and I went home and thought about how to tell Dr. Barrows that Dr. Manson was not sure the hemangioma was still there. Trying not to let the anger rip through our doctor-patient relationship, I took out a piece of paper so I would have a chance to read the words I would say, reread them, and tone them down. I did not want to call up and say the first words that came to mind: How could you even think of operating again, when you did not know if it was there? How could you have gone in a second time, been the executor of such major trauma, been responsible for all the risks involved if nothing was there? What kind of mistake is that for someone to make? Someone with your experience?

The only aspect of the future that was certain was that uncertainty would prevail. No one knew whether a second operation would be necessary. No one knew when we would know. An indefinite plan of periodic MRI brain scans was initiated. The MRIs would be performed until it was clear that either the hemangioma was still there or it was not, but no one was even sure how they would recognize that the time of clarity had come.

The doctor-patient relationship is commonly portrayed in popular television shows and movies as if the doctor is a tour guide leading a traveler down a well-mapped road to a predictable destination. In truth, often doctor and patient are walking together in the darkness with neither the route nor the destination visible; their open eyes enabling them to make out only shadows.

Gradually, I started to feel well enough to watch some daytime television. (It's pretty pitiful that that was mental progress.) The programs were peppered with advertisements for malpractice attorneys. Often several firms would advertise on the same television show, with ads repeating and competing during the same half hour: "Has your doctor hurt you?" an attorney would ask. "Could you be the victim of medical malpractice?"

I had thought that I knew I would never sue. After all, I was a doctor and I knew all the problems with malpractice suits in this country. But after I had heard the ads more than a hundred times, they started to work as they are designed to, first at an unconscious level and then at a conscious one, their message fueled by the seeming futility of my position.

Dr. Barrows had been right to be surprised in the hospital that I was not angry at him. When my anger did finally come out during the weeks following the surgery, what kept me from taking it out on him and from trying to take advantage of the millions of dollars that the television malpractice attorneys promised was simply his caring.

But my father had never met him and he seethed with anger. He wanted desperately to sue Dr. Barrows in order to get even. He did not tell me that until a year later, though, because he was worried that a lawsuit would hurt me permanently by making me think of myself as damaged goods. My father is still angry years later. In his own words, he was angry at Dr. Barrows for "having too much confidence in his skills and much too little concern for the effects of his actions on his patient or other people. The image is of somebody driving a car at ninety miles per hour through a small shopping center with a speed limit of twenty-five miles per hour, saying, 'I am the greatest driver in the world,' and then killing a child."

Weeks passed, and still I could not find even common words needed to complete a sentence. The numbing fatigue that meant even a brief conversation cost a half-day's rest was still present. I still could not stand up for any duration or walk for any distance without my blood pressure dropping too dramatically to sustain consciousness.

Matters continued to be made worse by not knowing how long the disabilities would last or which ones would be permanent, and by doubting how long friends and family would stay by my side. The doubts were engendered not by loved ones, who could not have been more constant, but by my own loss of self-worth, compounded by a growing awareness of how society sees

the differently abled, regardless of which name is used —
"crippled" or "handicapped" or "disabled" or "challenged."

When I was in school, I used to pray at night to be
granted a productive life. In my heart, behind the words were
dreams of accomplishing a single major identifiable work,
whether it was building a health care program or writing about
how groups of people could begin to live in peace together.
Now, I no longer dreamed, and my prayers changed. The old
ones troubled me; they teased me with their seeming impossibility. Now, I prayed that I might learn to measure successes
and failures in daily life, to touch other people's lives, and to
make the world a better place through small daily actions.

It was patients, not physicians, who gave me faith again
in the future, patients who had a realistic view of recovery.
Friends who had once been sick or had had surgery recounted
stories to me, stories never told in medical school, about
problems physicians do not discuss. Hearing about illness and
recovery from friends who had been patients, hearing truths
that matched my own experience, hearing both their trials
and their triumphs, enabled me to hope again. They spoke of
how long it takes to want to eat again, how long it takes to be
able to sleep at night and be awake during the day, how long
it takes to be able to go out the door alone without being
afraid — afraid of falling, afraid of getting sick, afraid of not
being able to make it back to the front door. They told stories
that even residents, spending a hundred hours a week in the
midst of patients' hospital care, do not hear, because they are
the stories that take place after patients go home.

Evelyn, an older colleague, called. She spoke of the
"mothballs" and "moldy spots" in her brain after her surgery.
She had had abdominal, not brain, surgery, but she still had
had a great deal of difficulty concentrating for more than four
months after the surgery. To say Evelyn is not a complainer

is like saying Genghis Khan was not a liberal. Once, sick with pneumonia, Evelyn had to crawl on hands and knees to get a bottle ready for her baby, dress the toddlers in their winter coats, and instruct them on how to get to the neighbor's house. Evelyn survives struggles and rarely refers to them. Yet the "mothballs and moldy spots" had been bad enough for her to raise decades later.

Ruth talked about the head injury she had suffered while hiking, and how it took her a year to return to medical school. The hardest task was learning to sort out information again; holding a conversation while background music was playing remained difficult for her even a year and a half after the accident.

Beth spoke with candor about her multiple sclerosis, with which she was diagnosed while completing medical school. Multiple sclerosis is a degenerative neurologic disease in which patients get progressively more physically disabled and may die when they can no longer move enough of their muscles to breathe. Beth takes no pity on herself, and I had heard her talk of her setbacks only twice, in the privacy of her home. She spoke more freely now, sensing that I would understand her illness in a new way. She spoke of the loneliness of being home sick and of the depression caused by not being able to take care of family members or do any work for stretches of time. These were words that now vibrated on the strings of my soul. She also spoke about how differently she feels now on days when she can work well than she did before she developed multiple sclerosis. We both understood how such days made it possible to forget about present and future disabilities, how all of a sudden we felt as if we could fly.

Some of the people who came to visit were people I had not known well before but who made extraordinary efforts to provide support. Ken was one. When he heard through the grapevine of my seizure and surgery, he called immediately. He wanted to come from New York to visit. The afternoon he arrived, we talked for hours about his experience living with diseases that dissipate but do not disappear.

He had had pancreatic cancer in high school, one of the cancers with the lowest survival rates. During his senior year, he tried to go to school in between chemotherapy sessions and against his doctor's advice. He was able to attend school for only seventy days, but was still able to graduate by reading at home. He said he had felt angry and guilty because of the pain that his illness had caused his family and friends, so at first he did not apply to college. By now, he had gone through college and graduate school. He did not talk about his recovery of a rich and meaningful life—ongoing uncertainty made that discussion too painful—but he demonstrated it. He was working as an advocate for the poor. He was a living reminder of the meaningful life one can lead at the end of a long illness, and a refreshing drink of hope.

On my kitchen table was an eight-and-a-half-by-eleven-inch paper filled with scrawled handwriting, a check-off list for the medicines to be taken each day. There were more than thirty pills to take, some twice a day, some three times a day, some four times a day. The pharmacy did not have a pillbox large enough for all the daily doses.

Dilantin was among the medications. Its purpose was to prevent further seizures that might occur as a result of the hemangioma—its original bleed, ongoing bleeding if it was still in my brain, or scarring from the surgery. Most medications exhibit a variety of side effects, different ones in different people. For weeks while taking Dilantin, I struggled to sit up or stand for long. In order to maintain consciousness when sitting or standing, the body needs sufficient blood pressure to move oxygen to the brain. My blood pressure was too low on Dilantin.

Dr. Barrows understood the disabling side effects of the Dilantin. "Stop taking the Dilantin for two days and then take half the original dose for a day and then you can stop altogether," he advised as soon as my Tegretol level was sufficiently high. Within a day the dizziness had dissipated. For the first time in weeks, I could sit up and read.

Dr. Barrows's attention to side effects continued when it came to stopping the steroids, although stopping them was not so easy. Steroids had been prescribed to limit the brain swelling that occurs after surgery. Dr. Barrows warned, "A lot of people have mood swings when they stop the steroids. You may feel very depressed. Don't worry, though; it'll go away within a week or so."

The language of physicians is usually filled with euphemisms. As a patient, I heard many of the same ones I had heard in medical school. "You may feel a little warmth" described the burning of a dye injection into the brain during an arteriogram. "You'll feel a little prick" described the large bore needle entering the groin. "You'll be uncomfortable for a few days after surgery" described uncontrollable pain. Dr. Barrows's honesty, his willingness to say "very depressed," contrasted sharply with the typical euphemisms.

I had no idea what chemically induced depression was until I stopped the steroids. I would be sitting at the kitchen table, and suddenly my mind would be flooded with thoughts of death: lying in bed, again thoughts of death, walking to the bathroom, all of a sudden overcome with sadness. Yet, I knew, intellectually, there was nothing I was newly upset about. The sudden depression was timed so closely to the stopping of the steroids that it was clear what was going on.

Even knowing the cause, the depression was uncontrollable. When the clouds of death came, I could say, "This is withdrawal," but the rain still poured. As Dr. Barrows had predicted, it lasted less than a week. Dr. Barrows's honesty made the whole process bearable.

Despite his mistakes, Dr. Barrows was an exemplary physician in most ways. He eased the pain of many transitions with his warnings. Even before the surgery, when he anticipated it would only take an hour and a half, he advised that it would be six weeks before I would begin to feel able to work again. He was the only physician among the many with whom Tim and I spoke who even hinted at the process of recovery that takes place at home. Dr. Barrows had himself spent weeks in bed as a patient, recovering from an injury. That experience contributed to both his concern and his understanding.

When there were setbacks in the recovery period, he often offered a rope to pull me out of the quicksand, saying, "I think you'll be feeling a lot better within two weeks." He started each conversation asking, "How are you feeling?" and he really wanted to know the answer. He made it clear that he was always available to answer questions and respond to concerns.

As I began to get better, I had lots of time to think about how lucky I was, time torn from work by the requirements of recovery.

AUGUST 14

We frequently observe the world of the elderly narrowing — reading less, having fewer outside interests. Yet, should it be such a surprise?

While laid up in bed, I have thought a lot about what the elderly have to deal with when they are sick, . . . how many times harder it must be than what I face. Many of their words — difficult to understand in the past as a grandchild or young physician on the wards — have returned, ringing in my ears.

Those facing new chronic disabilities are asked when they
are sickest and most fatigued to try and find the resources to
change, to learn, to adapt to that disability. With progressive
diseases and with progressive age, they may not have the
chance to wait until they are feeling better to adapt. When we
ask them not to accept defeat, do we understand the price of
victory?

When sick and exhausted, their time to be active is so
limited that they must choose their priorities. To the outside,
they are less interested in world events — maybe there is some
truth in that. As the texture of time changes, and there is little
they can do to affect world events, there is the realization that
world events will come and go on in dramatic ways long after
each of our lives, whose time is transparently brief.

It is only the hope of having a time in the future to look
forward to, a time when I will be able to be free of much of this
pain and the extreme degree of mental fatigue, that keeps me
trying to push my limits. Dreams of the future help keep me
writing in case the writing may help others one day. Dreams
help keep me reading about health and poverty programs and
international issues during the few minutes of concentration I
can muster each day. Dreams that one day I will be able to do
things for my family and friends again, to share more equally in
activities and responsibilities, keeps us going.

Even with dreams, sheer exhaustion and the limitations
on my mental alertness make the world narrower. Reading the
newspaper in detail would mean no other activities that day: no
writing, no visiting, no reading. Dreams of the future have the
power to brilliantly, if sporadically, illuminate the present like
fireworks on a moonless night.

In mid-August, Tim, Ben and I went across the street to
an open field for the first time since the surgery. I could not
believe how exciting it was to be outside, walking around the
field, the sun streaming down, watching Ben run. Despite

dealing daily with disease at work, how often had I taken such joys for granted? Would I ever take them for granted again? My father wrote after the surgery, "Jody and Tim will never be young again. I fear life will never feel like something to be trusted by them." He was right that the change was permanent but wrong to fear it would impoverish our lives.

Finishing the first lap around the field exhausted, I wondered, Should I do it again? Tim and I discussed it. Another lap or just a few more feet and then back home. I wanted to keep going to build strength. Tim rightfully reminded me of the number of times I had already overdone it. We both wondered how far is far enough to speed the slow process of recovering strength and rebuilding muscles? How far is too far? I walked around the field again. I could not resist.

It is rather remarkable that people talk about the road to recovery as if the path to take were well marked, the proper speed clearly indicated, and cars constantly traveling on it in one direction. That was neither my experience nor that of most people I know. Recovery was closer to a maze, with no road signs, a lot of false starts, a number of dead ends, and a great deal of backtracking before reaching any destinations.

My days at home were spent alone after my father and Danny left. My physical abilities had progressed a step at a time: first able to sleep alone quietly; then able to have short conversations; then able to jot down notes for minutes at a time; then able to read one page, then two; then able to hold longer conversations; then able to read for half an hour at a time and write a full page; then gradually able to sit up and free my hands for work; and then, several weeks later, able to take occasional accompanied excursions outside.

My appetite for work was voracious. As soon as I could sit regularly, my blood pressure having returned to normal, I went back to work with the wonder of a child's eyes at first seeing the ocean: it was huge and unfathomable, but I was so happy to be there to soak it in. My uncle Jim had just written a book about epilepsy. After walking outside, my first project was reading the book and writing back comments at his request.

The words that I had lost use of began to return as I wrote to Uncle Jim. Somehow closing my eyes and focusing on where the words were stored brought them back. The mental exercise was invisible — how it worked was difficult to understand — but it was just as effective as walking was at bringing back atrophied leg muscles.

My next project was returning to articles I had been writing on international AIDS and trying to bring some of the pieces to completion. The reminders to work fast because life was transient and unpredictable were present every morning in the mirror. The right upper side of my face was gradually returning to life, but not in the way the surgeons had expected. The nerve on the right, damaged, never returned. Instead, the nerve to the left side of the face slowly took on more and more responsibility and began to make more of the right side of the face move.

Around this time, Joe Briar, who had advised me on my medical thesis, called and urged, "You will have plenty of time to work on AIDS. You have a lifetime ahead of you. I want you to do something like origami." In my heart, I did not feel it was wise to count on having a lifetime ahead of me. That difference in our views was pushing me to do as much as I could with every day of life I had. Still, I heard his message. Although I kept working, his words did work like a valve on a pressure cooker to release some of the tension that was building up to bring projects to a closure quickly.

Now that I was home alone, I could no longer sleep during the day, but I needed more than the seven or eight hours of sleep that I got with Tim at night. Fear of dying? Not of the process of dying. In part, it was fear of not being, of an eternity without feelings, thoughts, experiences, without those I love if there was no life after death. But most of all, the recurrent fear that kept me from sleeping during the day was a fear of dying without my life having made any difference in the world.

In learning to accept the early death of several friends in high school, I had made bargains with myself: to soak up the life of each moment as if it were my last and to do everything I could to work by the adage that we should render this world a better place when we leave it than when we came into it. That adage came back to haunt me. I had loved many people and believed they had felt my love. I had rejoiced in life — maybe this was what my father saw as my courage. Yet I worried about whether my life made any difference in the world. I had tried. I had been doing volunteer and community service work for almost two decades, since I was eleven years old. But I wasn't sure any of it had made a difference in the long run.

One can make a difference in different ways. I was not a wealthy philanthropist who could help other people by building a boat with my name on it. All I had had were shared dreams and efforts. Not wanting the impact of my life to disappear as fast as ripples in a pond, I prayed that there might be effects of my community work and that of my co-workers that would last.

After too many days without sleep, my mind, out of fatigue, was far beyond the weariness of every other night duty call which I had done working in the hospital. I lay in bed crazed with sadness but unable to cry, exhausted beyond explanation, unable to think in sentences let alone ideas. The exhaustion from fighting in a foreign territory full of rabid feelings was so complete. Raw terror, raw fear, raw sadness, raw loneliness, no words. Not only no words to say that were adequate but no words I could find for myself. Was this the step before raving madness? Was this the person in a dream who through clenched teeth cannot talk?

Tim came in. He held me, he helped lay me down. His physical presence helping to assure me that the abyss would be denied its lonely due that night.

Finally, the next morning, I began to dream again; I needed to. Langston Hughes's poetry spoke to me not in abstraction but in the cold reality of survival.

> *Hold fast to dreams*
> *For if dreams die*
> *Life is a broken winged bird*
> *That cannot fly.*

The dreams did not begin with details — I knew too little of what physical capabilities I would have — but with writing down on scraps of paper long-held values:

> More than anything, I would like to help with the process of decreasing the distance that people feel between themselves and others. Maybe by decreasing that distance, we can get further toward caring enough as a society to ensure that human rights are respected. If we could decrease that distance we put between ourselves and those in other communities, maybe then we could truly become part of a world community, caring as much about what happens to others struggling for a full life at home and abroad as in our neighborhood.

By 10 A.M., I was too exhausted to write or move around the apartment and sat down at the kitchen table to try and read. With the first page it became clear my eyes would not move from the left to the right. They could not read because they could not see one word following another. Shaken, I tried harder and harder but was unable to read: I did not know what to do. I looked around the apartment for an escape, but my eyes would see only straight ahead. Frightened, not knowing what it was, whether it was the beginning of a seizure, I went to lie down. Waking up two hours later, I could see again.

Was it a seizure? After some seizures, people sleep from the fatigue of the post-ictal period. Or a new neurological problem? The brain scan still showed a ring-enhancing lesion, something that looked like a bright doughnut, with a hole in it that should not have been there. I called Dr. Beauregard, a neurologist who began caring for me postoperatively. Dr. Wilford, who was covering her practice, answered the phone, "I don't have any idea what happened to your eyes. It doesn't sound like a seizure to me, but I don't know. Why don't you just wait and see what happens?"—a disquieting prescription of ignorance.

Tim and I were about to go away with Ben, my college roommate, Joyce, and her husband, Ethan. Joyce and I had met the first week of college. Eight years after graduation, still among our dearest friends, Joyce and Ethan had invited us to join them in a one-story, whitewashed wood cottage they had rented for a week on Cape Cod.

When we arrived, I was feeling awkward, self-conscious and depressed about how little I could do to help Joyce and Ethan with daily chores, like dishwashing. If I could have seen the future and known whether I would recover enough to reciprocate in years to come, I might have felt differently, but I was worried about re-establishing relationships as a seeming burden for others.

As we sat outside on the lawn overlooking fields of tall grass, Ben napped indoors, and Joyce and Ethan tried to push me for future plans. As only close friends with confidence in me could have done, they made me begin to dream in detail.

We talked about Tim and my continuing to work overseas

and the adaptations it would require. I broached my hope that my writing could in some small way help bridge the gap between different groups of people in the United States as well as between people in the United States and people abroad who never meet.

Wild dreams, but heartfelt. Like many others, I had spent years editing my dreams to keep only the probable. Surgery had suddenly silenced the hand of that editor. God places enough limitations. I would never again add any unnecessary ones.

After days of resting, we were outside one afternoon playing croquet. Requiring walking no farther than twenty feet, allowing sitting between turns, and consisting of little else but swinging at a sitting ball, croquet is the perfect sport for those recovering from physical injury. I was winning the first round, not counting one-year-old Ben, who carried his ball from wicket to wicket. Then I began to deteriorate rapidly, like Charley in *Flowers for Algernon.* I went from being able to play to not being able to hit the ball with my mallet, trying harder and harder with no success. I could not see the ball. I could see the ball when it was sitting still in one place, but when the ball moved, I could not see where it went. I did not know if it had gone through a wicket or not. I could not see anything that happened at the sides of my field of vision or anything that moved. It was like playing while wearing a blindfold.

Finally, I sat down on the grass. Holding back the tears, I thought, It's okay: there are still ways to work around this. It's just going to take some time to figure it out. It just means one more obstacle. I was trying to convince myself to have courage. I focused on the many people in the world who are dealt far harder hands yet never stop their work.

Joyce helped me inside — since I was unable to see as I walked — and called Dr. Barrows since I was unable to follow the numbers as they moved around the rotary phone. "Dr. Barrows, I'm having problems with my eyes," I said. "They seem to be working fine, but then, over the course of a few minutes, everything changes, and I cannot see anything that moves. I cannot see anything out of the sides of my eyes. I cannot move them enough to be able to read or to be able to walk."

In contrast to Dr. Wilford, Dr. Barrows showed his concern: "I don't know what it is yet, but we'll work together and find out. I'll call one of the ophthalmologists right away. We'll go back and look at the CAT scans with the neuroradiologists and look at where that lesion is." He took the step so critical to providing quality health care. He had faith in the patient's report of what she was experiencing and did not fall into the trap so common a part of the arrogance of modern medicine of believing that something doctors do not know how to explain must not exist.

The diagnosis came later that week from Dr. Beauregard. The problem was the Tegretol. An unusual side effect of the Tegretol is limiting extraocular movements. In order to be able to read, to follow movements, or to look at the sides of the room, the eyes have to be able to move. We depend on our eye movements for everything but seeing straight ahead. Nerves and muscles work together to enable the eyes to move. Even a horse with blinders is able to move its eyes up and down and side to side within the blinders to follow motion. The Tegretol had crippled my eye movements.

The solution was neither simple nor straightforward. My Tegretol level was barely at the bottom of the "therapeutic range," the range in which medications are effective but not toxic for the average patient. Decreasing the Tegretol would mean risking a return of seizures. Switching to Dilantin was not a good option because of the toxic drops in blood pressure I had suffered previously. Phenobarbital, a third anticonvulsant, was the most sedating of the three and thus might present equally troubling problems for work.

Dr. Beauregard wanted me to stay on Tegretol at the same dose despite the side effects. She dreaded the possibility of seizures more than I did. Tim had seen the seizure, heard me scream, and struggled to get me into the ambulance. My own experience had been far different. That first seizure itself had been easy. I had fallen asleep as usual at his side and did not remember anything until after the seizure. It was waking up disoriented, among strangers, separated from my family that had been awful.

Dr. Beauregard could sense that seizures did not yet hold any stigma for me or provoke fear, so she tried scare tactics. She resorted to the stories of the rare patients who had seizures while cooking and suffered severe burns. But far more real to me than the risk of seizures were the disabling side effects of treatment.

In medical school, we are trained to treat disease. We are less often taught the need to balance the beneficial with the detrimental consequences of treatment. We rarely discuss the fact that one patient may weigh the costs and benefits of a given treatment differently from another patient, and that as a result medical decisions need to be individualized.

Medical educators will say, "We teach that the elderly dying patient might not find chemotherapy worthwhile, whereas the young patient would value any chance at extending his life." But that is a far different approach. It is an approach that depends on stereotypes and categorizes how different demographic characteristics might affect values placed on treatment. Little time is devoted to how to work with patients making choices on an individual basis. Furthermore, discussions of patient preferences are often limited by a focus on dying patients or on settings where modern medicine is ineffective. The message is clear that whenever effective treatments are available, they should be used in young people at almost any cost.

In practice, doctors are well regarded by their peers if their patients are seizure-free, particularly their patients who have difficult seizure disorders. When a patient comes into the emergency room with an unexpected seizure, the assumption is that improper treatment by the doctor or "poor compliance" by the patient is at fault. The same questions are always raised: "Who is the doctor? Why weren't the seizures managed better?" Yet the same peers spend little time discussing these questions: How well were the physicians considering whether they are giving the right amount of medication? What impact is the medication having on the patient's life? Were physicians evaluating the side effects of the medicines?

The inadequacy of this approach in my case was well demonstrated by the disabling hypotension of Dilantin and the blinding effects of the Tegretol-induced ocular paralysis. Talking to Uncle Jim was refreshing. A famous pediatric neurologist who specializes in treating seizures, he believes that individual patients should be helped to make their own decisions, to balance the risks of having a seizure — from either taking less of a particular medication or stopping it altogether — against the problems they are having from taking that medication, the side effects it is causing, and the risks to a pregnancy. More radically, he departs from the common practice of medicine by recognizing that individuals feel differently about these decisions.

After speaking with Uncle Jim, I spoke again with Dr. Beauregard. She was nervous about cutting back on the amount of Tegretol, but she was willing to give it a try this one time.

When I decreased the dosage of Tegretol, the side effects diminished. I noticed the sun shining in the window through the trees; I could follow the beam of light with my eyes from the trees all the way to my bed. There is a Yiddish tale that expresses better than any other words how I felt:

> An impoverished man in a ghetto was stuck in a house much too small for his whole family, and everybody was fighting. They had little to eat and no room to sit. So they went to see the rabbi.
>
> "Rabbi, what do I do?" the man asked. "We are so crowded."
>
> And the rabbi asked, "Do you have chickens?"
>
> "Yes."
>
> "Well, take in your chickens," he replied.
>
> The family spent the week with the chickens, which were cluck, cluck, clucking. It was getting worse. Now the man had his sister, her family, his mother-in-law, his wife, seven children, and the chickens in the house. So he went back to the rabbi.
>
> "Rabbi, it has gotten even worse. Those chickens are clucking and leaving feathers all over. What should I do?"
>
> And the rabbi asked, "Do you have goats?"
>
> The man said, "Yes."
>
> "Bring the goats in," the rabbi instructed.
>
> The man looked horrified, but he listened to his rabbi, and he brought the goats in. So now, the goats were running around the one-room house and urinating all over the floors and battering the little furniture he had. The chickens were still leaving their feathers all over and clucking. The family was fighting even more. He went back to his rabbi in desperation.
>
> "Rabbi, you cannot believe how much worse it is. What should I do?"
>
> And the rabbi asked, "Do you have a cow?"
>
> And the man did not want to answer truthfully, but he did: "Yes."
>
> The rabbi said, "Bring the cow into the house."
>
> The man did not believe it could get worse, but it did.

Now, on top of everything else, the cow was lying on their few pieces of furniture and breaking them. The children, instead of lying next to each other squeezed into a bed, were lying piled on top of each other at night.

Another week passed, and the man went back to the rabbi. He said, "Rabbi, I cannot take it anymore. I cannot help my sister and give her a house; we have no room. My mother-in-law and I — the fights are so bad that my wife is threatening to leave.

And the rabbi said, "Take the cow out."

And the man came back a week later and said, "You know, Rabbi, things are a lot better now."

Then the rabbi said, "Then take the goat out."

And the man came back joyous at what a beautiful home he had, and the rabbi said, "Take the chickens out."

By the end of that week, the man felt like the luckiest man on earth.

By the middle of September, so did I.

CHAPTER FIVE

The Wrong Side of the Fence

IN JULY, Dr. Weissman, the physician-in-chief at Children's Hospital had written:

> Dear Jody,
>   I have heard about all the plans and I am glad to know that a curative program is now in progress. Just remember that we are anxious only for your full recovery and look forward to working with you. Do not worry about it. Your place is here whenever you can make it. All the best.
>   Sincerely,
>   David Weissman

The letter took extra weeks to arrive because it had been sent to the wrong address, but the message stayed with me. In mid-September, I called up Dr. Weissman's office to set up an appointment to discuss coming back. The morning of the appointment, I dressed up in a skirt, stockings, and pumps. I washed my hair, wanting everything on the outside to look as ready to return as my heart felt. Dr. Weissman extended as warm a welcome as imaginable. I was near tears at the joy of being there but recognized crying might not be perceived as a power entry. Wrinkling his forehead and lowering his voice, Dr. Weissman asked, "But are you physically up to coming back? I don't want you back before you're ready."

"Yes, I'm up for it. I'm ready and doing things all day now at home. I'm taking care of Ben throughout the day, and I don't think there is anything much more exhausting than taking care of a one-year-old baby."

"Are you doing any running?"

Repressing laughter, I said, "No, but I never was a runner." The laughter came from the knowledge that I was a long way from running a marathon. It had taken all my strength to come this far.

Dr. Weissman and I, along with Renee, the chief resident, who oversaw all the interns and residents, set up a schedule. I would start at the end of September. The first month would begin with half days in the emergency room and build up to full days. By the end of October I would be working forty- to fifty-hour weeks but without "on call," overnight work in the hospital. The second month would increase toward sixty-hour weeks, again without "on call" work. At the end of two months, I would begin night call and ninety-hour weeks.

The realistic schedule was developed in large part due to Renee's own experience. As a resident, Renee had needed emergency surgery. Initially, she had viewed her recovery period with as little understanding as medical training provides. She assumed she would be able to go back to work full-time from the start. For the first time in her career, she "failed." Willpower was not enough to overcome her own unrealistic expectations. Mortified, she had been forced to cut back on her schedule. Medical school, residency training, and her own physician caregivers and supervisors had left her ignorant of the reality of recovery, but experience did not.

The program directors at Children's Hospital had had

some difficult experiences with residents who had returned after surgery. They were concerned about having difficulties with me too. But Dr. Weissman explained, "Some of our best physicians have come from past gambles." I owe a deep debt to the Children's Hospital Pediatric Department for being willing to give me a try. With that gamble, they may have saved more than one life; they certainly saved mine.

Renee urged me to come to the house-staff retreat in mid-September before starting internship. As I walked into the room of seventy house staff and recognized only one or two people, I felt the awkwardness of an adolescent who has moved to a new high school where all the other students know each other and are sitting with their friends. Dr. Weissman opened the meeting: "The first thing I would like to do is give a special welcome to Jody Heymann and to let her know how glad we all are that she's joining us." Nothing could have been a nicer gift at that moment.

He went on to talk about how the hospital was doing and what contributions, economic and human, the house staff made to it. "The hospital depends on the house staff, greatly. Your work as pediatricians on the neurologic service is critical. Neurosurgery makes a great deal of money for the hospital."

Suddenly, I sat there alone again, thinking of the $20,000 in hospital bills from my surgical admission. The impact of health care costs had never been more real. I was lucky. I had health insurance that covered most of the bills. I had disability insurance, which paid for half of my absence, until I was able to return to work.

While I had been recovering from surgery, a wood carver whom I had met on the street had not been so fortunate. He sat at a table with his carvings and a sign declaring his health care problems. He had $30,000 in hospital bills as the result of an accident. He had been making too little money before the accident to afford health insurance premiums — $4,000 a year as a self-employed person — like forty million Americans, he had had no health insurance.

As I sat in the crowded room of physicians, I heard less and less of what Dr. Weissman was saying. My thoughts were on health care costs, what they meant to patients as well as physicians, and what could be done for those patients who are uninsured or underinsured. The rest of the day I tried to pay better attention to relearning the hospital's perspective on the health care system. That house-staff retreat was both a celebration of renewal and a leveling shock.

On a crisp September Monday, soon after the retreat, I walked into the emergency room at 8:00 A.M. for my first day as an intern with as much eager anticipation and as little anxiety as I can ever remember having when starting a job. I knew how hard residencies were. But any concerns had been overtaken by relief at being well enough to return to work; I was grateful.

Children's Hospital had built a new, brightly lit emergency department. There, clean white walls cloak each child's sickness in a private room. Patients' status is reported and updated on the board at the front, which lists the names of the children who are in each room. Each room has its own significance. Room 15 is the gynecologic room, often occupied by a pregnant teenager or a child who may have been abused or raped. Room 29 is the urgent medical room. Room 30 is for trauma patients and patients who are "coding," that is, those who cannot breathe or whose hearts have stopped. The other rooms are for everyone from children with tumors who are coming in for their last hospital stay to children with a cold who end up in the emergency room for primary care because they have no regular doctor. That morning the board was clear, and there was no one in the waiting room.

Each Monday in the emergency department started with a conference at which residents presented to more senior physicians the case histories of patients they saw the week before. Mark gave the first presentation. He was clean-shaven, and his hair was still wet from a shower. He had come in from a good night's sleep at home instead of brief naps snatched while working overnight in the hospital.

Mark began, concealing the name of the patient, as was customary: "X was a fifteen-year-old boy who was in a car accident. By the time he arrived at the emergency department, he had lost a quarter of his blood and had multiple skull fractures; his squash was really fried." Phrases from the rest of his description came in and out of my mind in waves broken by the replaying of "his squash was really fried." To Mark it meant, Well, there was not much we could do for this patient's brain, so we really did not have to care about what happened.

Mark's words were not unusual. Physicians use jokes and coarse language to distance themselves from patients, to ease the difficulty of dealing with death, which does not look as clean or pretty in real life as it does on television, and to keep from feeling the pain of witnessing the destruction of the young and the devastation of the old. To make that task easier, the language is purposely dehumanizing. The doctor-patient relationship is an accidental casualty. I had tried to be an imperfect exception to the trend even before getting sick. I went lighter on the language by nature, but it would be ridiculous to pretend I had never made crass jokes. Students enter medical school caring about other people and identifying with their patients. Medical school does not stop them from caring, but it does try to shift their identification to one with the doctor.

We went on to the next case. John, another resident, sat in his mismatched scrubs. He had been working the previous night and the day before. By the time the emergency department settled down enough for him to change out of his street clothes into scrubs for the night, only one green extra-large shirt and tight blue medium pair of pants were left. John began telling a story of a teenager who came in with an overdose of drugs. "You can give Ipecac to adults who have overdosed to make them throw up a lot, if you want, but it's just to punish them," he explained, angry at the patients who seemingly contributed to their own illness. He knew there were better ways to treat overdoses. It was confusing to me to identify more strongly with the patients in the stories than the doctors, who were my peers.

Silently, I went about my work, going to the board, signing up for a number and name, and then walking instantly into the life of one family after another at their most vulnerable moments. I went into the orthopedics room of the emergency department, where Jerid lay on a gurney. The cause of Jerid's pain was obvious even before he sat down at the triage desk. The part of his arm that should have run straight from his elbow to his wrist was bent and broken. His X rays were falling out of the basket on the door. His arm was in a sling, and he was screaming and crying in a panic. From down the hall, we had all heard the screams. He was barely three years old.

"Hi, Jerid. Your arm must really hurt. I promise I won't touch it without telling you." He began to look up through his sobs. "First, I just want to sit and talk to you and your mommy and hear what happened." Then, after pausing, "It's been such a bad night for you, and you've been so brave." His sobs were subsiding as I kept talking, explaining quietly again that I would not touch or do anything to him without telling him first, and gently again that I understood how much it hurt. Gradually, when I had been there long enough without doing anything that had hurt him, he ceased his warning cry.

Jerid embodied the interplay between fear and pain. His

arm was broken and throbbing. Having an intravenous line placed for medications and getting his arm set would be painful. But the worst part for him was fear of the unknown, compounded by lack of control over grown-ups who would hurt him. He had come to the hospital to get better and immediately was hurt and scared by a rapid sequence of diagnostic procedures that involved movements of his already excruciatingly pained arm. No one told him what would come next. The brightly lit hospital seemed more like a house of horrors in the shadows.

As grownups, we have a whole set of expectations about the world that young children do not share. Two years later, when Ben was Jerid's age, he and I went to a train museum together. I thought he would be overjoyed. In fact, he was terrified by the large trains. Finally, he explained he was afraid they would run him over. It had never occurred to me that the adult assumption, that large trains parked in a museum do not move, was a learned one.

At the hospital, everyone who examined Jerid and took X rays did so to help him. But each procedure caused him pain, and Jerid did not know whether to expect the next person to do worse. As soon as he knew he would be told about everything before it happened, as soon as his pain was acknowledged and he was given time to gather himself together, his demeanor changed completely. Jerid was remarkable, not for his response to fear of pain and of the unknown but for his ability to accept procedures that hurt once he was told what would happen.

As soon as Jerid had ceased crying, I took the history of the accident, beginning with his story, expanded upon by his mother. He looked into my eyes as he told me what happened. With broken limbs, one of the most important parts of the physical exam is to ascertain that neither the nerves nor the blood vessels have been severed by the break. Jerid began to smile with pride as he accomplished pieces of the neurologic exam by moving each finger in turn. His neurovascular system was intact. His X ray told the rest of the story: his forearm was broken in two places. There was no reason to conduct the painful parts of the exam before giving him painkilling medication. Analgesia would be necessary to set his broken bones.

The orthopedist requested I place an intravenous line in his intact arm. Knowing the intravenous line was necessary for pain relief but worried and sad that inserting the needle intravenously would bring back Jerid's wailing fearful cries, I began to explain quietly.

"Jerid, I need to put a special piece of plastic in your arm to give you medicine. It'll hurt for a minute when I put it in, but then the ouchy is over, and the medicine will keep your arm from hurting."

Lying amid buckets of water and rolls of powdery casting strips, he did not budge or cry while the intravenous line was placed. On equal footing, nursed with truth and patience, he showed a strength bordering on stoicism.

Caitlin was eighteen. She lay trembling on the stretcher, in clothes she had hastily thrown on. Her cerebral palsy made her movements awkward. Developmental delay had affected her speech, but she was able to live independently of her family in a sheltered setting.

She came alone by ambulance. She explained she had had seizures in bed. She had run out of her anticonvulsant medicine, Tegretol, two days before. She had described the seizures to a resident the night before.

"My whole body was shaking like this," she said, while demonstrating with her left arm and leg, which had been hanging limply off the stretcher. "I was awake, but I couldn't stop it."

This was not the kind of seizure that Paul, the resident caring for her the night before was used to hearing about. More commonly, patients are not conscious when their whole body is seizing with tonic clonic movements. He did not know what she was describing. More important, he made the mistake of not admitting to himself or to her that he did not know what she was talking about. He told her that nothing was the matter, that shaking like that could not possibly have been a seizure, and sent her home.

When she returned to the emergency department the next morning, I signed up for her on the board. The attending came to warn me: "She may be a difficult patient. She was swearing at the resident last night."

When I walked into her room, she was in tears. "No one believes me, no one believes me. They sent me home, and I had more seizures."

She described the seizures, which began with contractions in her right arm and spread to her left arm. Within seconds, both arms and both legs shook uncontrollably. This continued for minutes while she lay awake, alone and terrified, in bed. She felt violated. She had come to the hospital for help, and she had been sent home without medicine, only to have it happen again. This time, she came in even more terrified and upset. Of course she had been swearing; of course she had been "difficult." She had not received the care she needed.

"Why wouldn't they just give me some Tegretol until the pharmacy opened, so that this wouldn't happen to me again?" she asked with exasperation in her voice. She had come to the only place she knew would have medicine in the middle of the night.

"I believe you. I believe that what you're saying happened did happen. We'll figure out together what it was and how best to treat it."

"It was a seizure — I just need the Tegretol," she continued.

I knew little more than the junior resident the night before about whether or not she had had a seizure. But I did not doubt her terror; I could tell from her face that something had happened. It was better to err on the side of believing patients. I called her neurologist to find out if this was typical of her seizures, and in fact it was. She had partial complex seizures. This was exactly what happened every time. She never swore at me; she was never "difficult." She received her Tegretol in the amount recommended by her neurologist. She went home, leaving me to wonder how often we all undervalue the statement of another human being's experience, and to worry that I could make the same mistake.

Of all the hospitals in which I had been a patient, a family member, a medical student, or a physician, none was better than Children's. I saw many patients in the emergency department who received outstanding care. Still, there were repeated reminders of how medical education and the finances and organization of medical care in the United States affect our doctor-patient relationships and leave patients' voices unheard.

When I met Jane's mother in the emergency room, she was worried about whether there was any treatment for Jane's neck pain. The prolonged, severe neck pain was interfering with both Jane's junior high school attendance and her activities outside school. Jane seemed to have decreased strength on physical exam. At the end of the exam, I explained, "I don't know what's causing the pain, but we're going to do a complete workup to try and find out; I know the pain is real," I added, because I had begun to learn how often patients' experiences are doubted. The words seemed obvious and simple.

Her mother began to cry. It had been a long time since anyone had taken Jane and her mother seriously. Jane had been going to emergency rooms and doctors' offices for years complaining of neck pain, and no one could find the cause. As professionals too often do, they began to disbelieve what they could not understand.

The neurology resident came to evaluate Jane. Afterward, he pointed out inconsistencies he believed he had found in her exam and said he was sure she was faking her weakness. I did not know what to think anymore. I knew the neurology resident had a great deal more experience than I did with neurologic exams and conditions; that is why I had asked for his advice. Moreover, I had been taught in medical school about patients who fake symptoms. Still, I believed her pain and pushed for further care for her.

Three days later, as I walked out of the emergency department, Jane's mother stopped me. Magnetic resonance imaging had found the problem at last. Neck muscle abnormalities were pulling Jane's cervical spine out of alignment. The physicians caring for her did not yet fully understand what was going on, but once there was visible radiologic evidence, they all began to treat the problem as real. But it had always been real for Jane and her family.

As residents, we each had a clinic day. Throughout the year, we would leave our rotation once a week to spend the afternoon seeing outpatients. Children would come in for routine visits, vaccinations, and acute and chronic health problems.

Karl had recently immigrated from Russia. For his first physical he arrived with his mother, his sister, a Russian translator, immigration forms, and vaccination records from Russia. After hearing in translation an uneventful abbreviated medical history, I began to ask the standard "review of systems" questions.

"Have you had any headaches?"

"No."

"Any problems with your ears? Your eyes? Your nose? Your throat?" I asked, pointing to each body part. Karl and his mother shook their heads no, often before the translator had time to translate each item into Russian.

"Any vomiting or diarrhea?" I asked, pointing to his stomach.

"Yes, vomiting," Karl's mother answered, this time waiting for the translation to make sure she understood.

"How long have you had vomiting?" I asked, expecting that the problem might have lasted a few weeks at the longest without medical attention.

He was silent, and his mother answered, "About three years."

"Has he ever seen a doctor about it?" I asked, no longer knowing what to expect.

"Yes. They did some tests and told us it was not serious." The physicians had done nothing while Karl kept vomiting for three years.

How could his vomiting have been ignored for so long in Russia? The same way as it could have been ignored in the United States. The doctors ruled out anything they considered serious, any underlying disease that was potentially life-threatening or disabling as they defined it. What they ignored was that the symptoms were seriously affecting their patient's life over an extended period of time. They may have ignored the symptoms for any of the inadequate reasons health care professionals here could have ignored them — disbelieving Karl, labeling his symptoms psychosomatic, not knowing what his symptoms were from or how to treat them.

Under the supervision of the clinic attendings, I ran tests to determine that Karl had no life-threatening underlying illness. When that had been ruled out, I asked other physicians if it could possibly be due to chronic constipation. Dr. Jensen had discussed several cases of children he had seen at Children's Hospital who were so constipated that their intestines "backed up" and some food was regurgitated as vomit. We started Karl on mineral oil, an innocuous over-the-counter remedy for constipation.

Within weeks the vomiting was gone for good. Months later the Russian translator told me that the family had begun to call me a "white witch" because of the "magic" I had worked. There had been no magic except for taking seriously what the boy and his mother reported, believing that he had vomited on and off for years, and feeling with them that three years of even intermittent vomiting had a serious effect on his life and required attention.

By mid-October, I was slowly regaining strength while working half days. My thirtieth birthday was the first night in four months Tim and I tried to go out alone without Ben. Ben went to visit my parents, who had given us tickets to the local repertory theater. I was feeling a little sick. Getting sick is common for residents who work in a pediatric emergency department; many of the children with whom residents come into contact are vomiting, or have diarrhea, sniffles, coughs, or more. Working in the emergency department, after the immunosuppressant course of steroids had temporarily decreased my ability to fight off infections, made me a setup.

Tim and I talked. "Let's go out anyway," I voted. "We've been planning this for so long. It'll be really fun."

We are each a complicated web of emotions. I was not eager to accept physical limitations. But there was something else that made me stupidly, stubbornly try to go out that night. Tim and I had pulled ourselves through some rough waters over the previous four months. Most of the time we had pulled together, but there had been times when our rowing was at odds with each other. Everything from the surgery to my inability to drive placed demands on our time and on our physical and emotional energy, which had already been stretched by having

two careers and a baby. We addressed the extra demands together by each giving 100 percent of what we were able instead
of the previous compromise of giving 50 percent of what was
needed. Somehow we had made it through the worst, and never
had I been more in love. The last thing I wanted to do was ruin
that moment of celebration and recuperation.

But after four trips to the bathroom during dinner, growing sick with the same scourge as the children I had been
treating — diarrhea and finally vomiting — even I knew I could
not make it through a play. We started back home on foot until
I was about to faint and sat down on the curb between two
cars.

"Just one minute, Tim. In maybe just a minute I'll be able
to get up. I just feel a little lightheaded. I'm sure I'll be able to
do fine."

Some people never learn, or at least they learn slowly.
Minutes passed. Each time I stood, the world became progressively darker, my mind went blank, and I was ready to faint.
Luckily, a musician played nearby for a sidewalk audience. As
Tim ran home to get the car, and I sat next to the street
listening to the music, my thoughts went over the past two
months and the joys of being strong enough now to go out,
even if it was just to hear a curbside musician.

OCTOBER 24

Worked a full day!

What a remarkable day, the first full day in four-and-a-
half months.

This was also the first day that enough forgiveness washed
into Ben's heart for him to open his arms as he had every day
before the surgery and to stand, expectantly calling, "Ma, Ma,
Ma, Ma," counting on me to be there to lift him off the ground
with love.

CHAPTER SIX

No Distance

Each MONTH, the residents rotate to a new ward service, face new problems, and try to handle new responsibilities. The rotation system is designed to cover the needs of the hospital while providing residents with as broad an exposure to medicine as possible. In November, I was assigned to the neonatal intensive care unit (NICU) at the Brigham and Women's Hospital in Boston. More than ten thousand babies are born each year at Brigham and Women's. The residents at Children's Hospital serve as pediatricians on call for the deliveries and care for sick newborns.

At the entrance to the NICU stand eight-by-six-foot carts filled with yellow gowns, pressed and clean, to be worn over street clothes. The carts are surrounded by laundry bags for soiled gowns, which are sterilized after each use. The procedure for entering the NICU is only slightly less aseptic than that for entering a surgical suite. There is a sink outside each ward, surgical scrub brushes, pedals to control the water so that faucets, which could contaminate the hands, need not be touched, and doors that can be opened by leaning into them, so touching knobs with hands is unnecessary.

The babies in the NICU are often one-fifth, and sometimes one-tenth, as big as regular newborns. Some are so small they can be held in the palm of their parent's hand. The youngest premies, with their elfin faces and differently proportioned bodies, look more like fetuses than full-term babies.

The babies are often unable to cry or communicate with sounds because a plastic endotracheal tube — a small plastic straw in the throat that brings life-sustaining oxygen to the immature lungs — blocks any vocal cord movement. They are often unable to lift their limbs, which are weighed down with tiny needles, plastic intravenous lines, and intraarterial lines held in place with miniature arm boards and the smallest available tape, which is still as large as the babies' thighs. The nurses spend their whole shift attending to one or two infants, providing urgent medical care, teaching new parents and new pediatricians how to love these fragile human beings, how to hold them, how to talk to them, how to sing to them, how to soothe them.

The newborns are attached by wires to sophisticated machines that count their respirations and heartbeats. The machines are supposed to sound an alarm only when a baby has ceased breathing or a heart has stopped beating. But often, the bells are set off by a baby's sudden and momentary exuberance, expressed in awkward unexpected movements.

My first week in the NICU was exciting. But it was also exhausting to begin my first full-time month since having surgery working in an intensive care unit. Although the anticonvulsant's side effects had diminished with changing medications and decreasing the dose, they remained very troubling. An hour and one-half after I took each dose, I felt increasing fatigue. I could work through the side effects, but the most marked effects followed the final dose each day at home; I worried that my time with Ben and Tim, already limited by internship, was being further exhausted by medications.

Doctors pay attention to the life-threatening and permanently disabling risks of medications. If they did not pay attention, they would be sued. And doctors warn patients, as they should, of these risks, even if the risks are rare. But often doctors say little or nothing to patients of the common side effects that degrade the quality of their lives. Those doctors who do want to describe side effects to patients may not be able to find adequate information. The standard reference, the *Physician's Desk Reference,* is a compendium of information on medications provided by drug companies; it provides a list of possible side effects — often scores of them for a single drug — with no information about how common the side effect is, how long it will last, or what can be done about it.

Dr. Beauregard felt strongly that I should take the Tegretol for at least a year before trying to decrease the dose further. But another physician had a different idea. At her hospital, anticonvulsants were given routinely for only three months post-op because surgery often successfully removed the source of seizures. Decisions were made on an individual basis. Given the side effects I was experiencing, she said, "I would have recommended a gradual tapering of the medication for you, and observation. You're not driving. You're not a cardiothoracic surgeon. There wouldn't be any real risk to you or to those you care for if you did have a seizure. If you have a seizure, you'd just need to go back on the medication." I sat between the two physicians, the out-of-town physician, whose beliefs more closely matched my feelings about the costs and benefits of taking medication, and my physician, who was not willing to take any chances but did not perceive the price I was paying for her caution.

I tried talking Dr. Beauregard into a general decrease in my medication, but she fervently disagreed. So, as countless patients before me and since, I became what doctors complain about and criticize, a noncompliant patient. I had been taking 400 mg a day of Tegretol and began to take half a pill less in the evening: 350 mg a day.

In medical language, *compliance* is defined as going along with what the doctor has decided is best for the patient to do. Doctors take it to mean that the patient is treating their disease "correctly." Doctors commonly talk about *noncompliance* as a way of blaming patients, as in "He had a bad attack of asthma because he was noncompliant." And that is supposed to say it all. It means, He did not agree to take the treatment, so he got what he deserved. Most physicians rarely talk about valid reasons that the patient might not have followed a physician's recommendations. Doctors cannot believe that there is ever a good reason for rejecting decisions they make alone on behalf of patients. Doctors do not consider that their patients may bring different values and life experiences to their decisions, or that they may weigh the risks and benefits of a particular course of action differently than physicians do.

Sometimes the strength of a physician's opposition to his patients' making independent choices is communicated directly, as when physicians threaten not to continue to take care of patients if they do not follow their advice. Sometimes, physicians' closed attitudes are communicated indirectly to patients, and patients understand that if they disagree strongly with the doctor or do not follow the doctor's recommendations, it will affect how they are treated. As a result, I have seen many people shy away from discussions with their physicians about their own reluctance to follow the advice given.

It is hard to communicate the strength of the stigma of

"noncompliance" except to say that of all the personal points in this story, of all the vulnerable moments, perhaps the hardest to share with the medical community is the week when I was noncompliant. I write about noncompliance here hesitantly but honestly, with the hope that this discussion will help further open the dialogue about what patient participation means. Many studies have shown that when patients are not actively involved in decision making, they end up doing what I did with the Tegretol when the side effects were affecting the quality of my life: more than half do not complete the prescribed treatment.

Each night I would leave the NICU happy from a full day of work but exhausted. Once home, I would rapidly fade with fatigue and lightheadedness. The evening would end with a headache. As I took less medication, the side effects of fatigue and lightheadedness began to lighten. I was filled with the anxious excitement of thinking maybe I would be able to start living with fewer side effects, but knowing that daily I was risking seizures.

One night, just after falling asleep, both of my arms and legs began to shake uncontrollably. As the muscular movements became more and more violent, I called to Tim, dazed from being abruptly woken.

"What's happening? . . . Hold me, Tim."

That was the last thing I could say. There was a horrible fraction of a second when in forced silence I felt the spread of the seizure from one part of my brain to the entire brain before losing consciousness. Coming to minutes later, I could barely move the left side of my body. I was terrified. In many ways, only Tim had lived through the first seizure; he was the only one who had witnessed it. It had been easy for me to face bravely the possibility of future seizures when I remembered nothing of the first one. One minute I was there; the next minute I was there again, waking up in the emergency room, disoriented and frightened, but the seizure itself was a blank. This one was totally different. This time I felt the terror that Caitlin had described in the emergency room: the terror of being awake while her body moved violently out of control of her mind.

The hemiparesis was new. When I woke up after the first seizure, in June, both arms and legs had worked fine. This time, I could barely lift my left leg. My left arm was weak. The left side of my face sagged.

The weakness was accompanied by the terrifying thoughts that physicians are privileged to have. Was this just part of the seizure, in which case it would be short-lived, or was it caused by a bleed? A bleed in the area where the hemangioma had apparently been left by the surgery could cause precisely these symptoms. If so, the symptoms could be permanent. (Anticonvulsants protect against seizures but not against bleeds.)

Tim was too much of a perpetual optimist and I was too tired to bother panicking. Every ten minutes I tried to do a little more with my left arm and leg. After two hours, I could lift my left leg off the floor, and it finally became clear that strength was returning. By the following morning, the weakness in my limbs was barely perceptible, and I went to work.

It would be the only seizure of the year about which there was not any fuss at work. There was no fuss because no one knew. No one noticed anything different while I was at work because there was nothing to notice. That evening I left work and went to Sinai for a CAT scan to rule out a bleed.

My brain was the same, but now there was a difference in my heart: I was afraid of the next seizure. I was not afraid of injury to myself or others. The seizure had done neither of those things. I was afraid of those minutes when my arms and legs would be moving increasingly violently out of the reach of my mind.

Dr. Beauregard recommended increasing my dose of medication slightly to 450 mg. This time, I did so willingly, knowing I had tried everything possible to decrease the side effects in order to increase the energy I had for ninety-hour work weeks in the hospital followed by parenting, and to increase the chance of having a teratogen-free pregnancy.

After a month of working in the NICU, I rotated to Team B, the ward service for adolescents, and began to be on call. Questions and problems are directed to the intern on call overnight when the other resident and attending physicians go home to sleep. The decisions interns need to make at night are the unanticipated ones. Sometimes they are trivial decisions that were not bothered with during the day but that require a physician's signature for legal reasons, such as a patient's request for aspirin. Often the nurses suggest an answer while asking a question. "What should we do about Jane's diarrhea? Normally, we would . . . Would you mind signing an order for . . ." At other times, the unanticipated decisions revolve around downturns and near disasters. The amount of backup available depends on the senior resident who is supervising. The resident may be sequestered far away or she may be constantly at the intern's side. How the resident handles her supervisory responsibility, her teaching duties, and the other demands placed on her simultaneously depends on her judgment.

During my first night on call on Team B, the resident had to supervise two interns: one on Team C and one on Team B. The resident was busy with Team C's intern, so I did not see her all night long. We spoke only once on the phone. Had there been a serious problem, she would have been available. In fact, there were many other residents in the hospital who would have been available in an emergency. The problem is always whether or not the intern or other junior person will recognize what is serious and request supervision. That ability takes training.

At the same time as I was exhilarated to begin to care for patients independently, I was terrified that I would have a seizure when I had to stay up most of the night on call. Fatigue can cause recurrent seizures, and extreme fatigue can even bring on first-time seizures. In the military, nights of sleep deprivation have been found to cause soldiers who have never had seizures in the past to have their first ones.

For any intern who gets sick on the job, an event that happens many times a year, there are backups. I knew there would be no problem for patients even if a seizure occurred; had that not been the case, I would not have continued to care for them. So why was I terrified? Because I did not know what prejudices people would have. If I did seize, would my internship be all over, at least for now? Would they decide I could not make it? Would I lose my job? Or would they understand that there was no practical difference between me and the intern who during the previous week had fainted on the job from diarrhea? Generalized seizures and fainting, both resulting in the sudden temporary loss of consciousness, had long been perceived differently. (The federal law that currently prohibits discrimination on the basis of disability had not yet been passed. Since the law's passage, enforcement remains partial.)

At 4:00 A.M., after taking care of all the sick patients on the floor that night, I went to rest. There was still time left to lie sleeplessly, wondering. If I did seize, would I be found? Or would I just discover myself on the floor? I would be sleeping alone in the on-call room, a hundred feet from the ward nursing desk.

I have never awakened more relieved than the next morning, when I realized that I had made it through the night.

On Team B, I took care of Mark and Janet at the same time. Both had been completely healthy children before they were suddenly struck with life-threatening illnesses and the possibility of neurological devastation.

Janet, a seventeen-year-old high school student, left soccer practice early one day. When her mother came home, Janet told her, "I have a headache." Then she added after a pause, "Maybe I'm a little sick, too." It did not seem to be anything out of the ordinary at first; Janet acted as if she had the flu. But within hours, she was unconscious and needed a machine to help her breathe. She could not speak for days. Meningococcal meningitis was diagnosed. She survived the intensive care unit stay without coagulopathy or SIADH, the medical terms, respectively, for the complications that can lead a patient to bleed to death or become fatally dehydrated.

When she was transferred from the intensive care unit to the regular adolescent ward, five days after she had first become sick, she was still unable to talk and unable to recognize her family. She could push herself only three inches off the bed on her hands. She was able to open her eyes only a third of the way if she strained. She would look straight ahead without any recognition, pain plastered on her silent face. Yet she had passed the worst part of the infection. The prognosis looked far better than she did.

When Janet lay devastated, I was scared to be too upbeat with the family, but that was when it mattered to them the most. This was one disease that Fran, the attending physician, had had enough experience with to make an educated guess about the prognosis. When I worried that too positive a prognosis could mislead the family unfairly, Fran reassured me, "I have treated dozens of cases like this. She is going to get totally better. Tell the family — it will make a big difference." Janet's mother and I sat and talked at the bedside as Janet lay unable to communicate. Uncertain what Janet could comprehend, I was relieved that I was there to share good news.

Janet was already on antibiotics. Each day Janet's mother and I would talk at length about what advances Janet had made and repeat the discussion of her encouraging long-term prognosis. After ten days, the change was miraculous. Janet was up and about, talking, walking around, and dressing herself.

This time, she looked better than she was. She still could not do simple math. As her physical abilities increased, so did her awareness of her new limitations. She sat in the bathtub trying to shampoo her hair, unaware that it was dry.

Before Janet's discharge, I told her mother that we were very optimistic about a complete recovery but could not know for a few weeks or months whether there would be small deficits. I was worried my words would ring hollow to a parent who wanted to make sure her child would be "perfect" again. I was wrong. She was so glad Janet was alive, walking, and recognizing her that she was prepared to deal with whatever came next.

Three months later, Janet's mother sent me a card; Janet had gone back to high school and was on her way to college.

Mark's first-grade teacher noticed him staring straight ahead. Then suddenly he vomited, fell back in his chair, and seized. His mother, the ambulance, and paramedics were at his side in minutes. Within moments of their arrival, Mark was blue, and a plastic tube was placed down his throat to assist his breathing. At Memorial Hospital, he was in status epilepticus, a state of constant seizures, for two hours. Status epilepticus itself has a 10 percent mortality rate for an acute episode. That does not include the risk of death the patient faces from whatever underlying disease is ravaging the body and mind. Mark was transported to the intensive care unit at Children's Hospital. He was so sick that he required a doctor, as well as the expertly trained emergency medical technicians, in the ambulance.

Five days later, breathing on his own but with mental status changes all too apparent, he was moved from the intensive care unit to Team B. At ten o'clock in the morning, he could not remember what he had had for breakfast. His arms and legs would intermittently shake and create dancelike movements beyond his control. Talking that first night on the ward with his mother was far harder than talking with Janet's mother. We went outside, where I could tell her the truth without fearing it would discourage Mark. I led her to the conference room, constantly in use during the day but empty at night, where she could break down without worrying about Mark's reaction.

Trying to start with what good news we had, I explained, "We're so glad to see him out of the ICU, doing so much better breathing on his own, getting up, walking about, improving every day."

"Will he get all the way better? . . . Will he be himself again? . . . Will he be the boy I had a week ago?" she asked, her speech halting, but her words direct.

"I don't know. I wish we knew and could tell you now, but the truth is we don't know. We don't know yet what caused this. It looks like a viral encephalitis, and children's experiences with viral encephalitis vary greatly. But the best thing we know right now is that he's getting better and he's improving every day."

It is always a tightrope walk trying to be realistic and reassuring when doctors often do not know an outcome with any certainty. There are statistics for some sicknesses; for many others there are not. What statistics do exist are usually quite general. They may indicate how many people survive a disease without disability but they will not say how many seven-year-olds who have encephalitis with mental status changes five days later have no long-term aftereffects. So doctors are often left guessing.

She broke down crying. I put my arm around her, wishing Mark would get all better, wishing I could honestly reassure her, and trying to hold back from crying too. Mark was sitting quietly in his first-grade class one minute and taking a roller-coaster ride through hell the next.

At a medical conference the next day, interns, residents, and attendings talked together about how to handle different situations. I raised the dilemmas involved in breaking mixed or bad news. Joel, a psychiatrist, talked about his experience in the neonatal intensive care unit. He said, "All the parents want to hear is that their baby's going to be perfectly normal. That's the one thing you can't tell them. Nothing else you say will ever be adequate, but at least you can be as honest as possible with them and let them know that you will be there by their side."

So I spent many hours over the days that followed hoping to substitute time with Mark's family for what the medical profession lacked in treatment and knowledge. We could treat Mark's seizures. We could help him through the crisis of status epilepticus. But we had no medication for the encephalitis.

Four days later, his mother came to me in intense excitement. Mark knew where he was; he knew he was in the hospital. Anxiously she asked again, in a voice pressured to control the fear, "How much will come back?"

Mark's father wanted to know whether he would be able to take Mark ice fishing, as they had planned, between Christmas and New Year's. He was bargaining: please don't let anything change.

Two weeks passed, and Mark continued to improve slowly. We were getting close to the point when we thought he could go home. Then, while we were beginning to make discharge plans, he developed vomiting and diarrhea. We hoped it was just the flu from his roommate.

We moved him to a private room, so he would not have to share the bathroom with another sick child. I walked into his new room at noon — I will never forget the time — to see Mark and his mother. She said merely, "He's not looking like himself." I looked down at him staring ahead and saw that he was clearly starting to have a seizure. "It's going to be okay. I'm just going to get a nurse." I went to the nursing station right across from his room and said, "Mark's beginning to seize. Can you get me some help, please?" in a hurried voice and went right back to his bedside. I was watching him to make sure he was having no difficulty with his breathing. I hoped this seizure would be short. After all, he was on two anticonvulsants. Status epilepticus is rare once a patient is on anticonvulsants, and Mark had been improving.

The senior resident rushed to the bedside. Together, we turned Mark on his side and padded the area around him with pillows to prevent him from aspirating vomit or hitting the bed's hard metal rails as he seized. We put airway equipment nearby in case he had trouble breathing. We put an oxygen mask over his face. The nurse pulled his mother, who was crying hysterically, from the room, sat her down in the hallway, and stayed with her.

The minutes ticked by. We drew blood gases from Mark's arm to see if he was getting enough oxygen. He did not stop seizing. We got a third and a fourth anticonvulsant medication and began to give them. The senior resident called for anesthesia and ICU backup. With backup present in case the medications caused Mark to stop breathing, we pushed additional anticonvulsants. Finally, the seizure stopped. Mark was on his way back to the ICU.

The episode was terrifying because it had been so unexpected. He was on treatment and he still went into status epilepticus. He could have been at home.

In the end, Mark did well. He soon returned to the Team B floor. His improvement was steady, and he was discharged home. His parents later told me that they could not sleep for the first weeks he was home. Worrying that he would go into status epilepticus again, they woke with every movement he made.

The day after Mark's seizure, one of the other interns working on Team B said to me as we were writing up patient reports, "It's so scary, someone like Janet, who'd been so healthy, getting meningitis. I know I won't get cystic fibrosis or hemophilia [congenital diseases affecting a number of children on the ward], but meningitis could happen to me. I can't imagine it."

I could not believe he had just said that. I guess I did not realize how much distance other interns still had. My nightmare was always the same: I would be working in a remote area of a developing country and I would go into status epilepticus. I would be unable to breathe, and there would be no one there to help. Status epilepticus is rare among those who have seizures, but one would never know it from the number of children I treated in status epilepticus. For patients who are in status epilepticus the mortality rate is high in the United States, and it would be astronomical in remote areas overseas.

For many residents, reminders of their own vulnerability are rare and frightening. For me, they were a part of daily life. The reminders changed the kind of doctor I was. There was a difficult patient on the ward at that time, diagnosed with both gastrointestinal disease and mental illness. He kept calling for whichever intern was on call, all night long, with one problem after another. After a night when I had gone in to see him half a dozen times, the patient's primary intern asked me why I kept answering his calls. Why did I not just go to sleep and tell the nurse not to wake me for them? The real reason was that in July I was a patient with aseptic meningitis, and the resident would not get out of bed. When I spent many extra hours with Janet's and Mark's worried families, I would often think about my family and how much support from physicians or its absence had meant to them.

Many residents, but by no means all, have built strong walls around themselves. They know they are past the threat of congenital diseases and they do not imagine they could have a child with a problem at birth. They often have no children, have never been seriously sick, have never worried about having a high-risk pregnancy themselves, do not see themselves as parents or as patients. They rarely have feared a lifetime of disability.

My walls had come tumbling down, and I did not want to rebuild them.

CHAPTER SEVEN

Code Blue

As INTERNS, we rotated through intensive care services and ward teams for different-aged children. My next rotation was Team C. Team C, designed for children older than the infants and toddlers of Team A and younger than the adolescents of Team B, often had children of all ages when another team had taken too many admissions or filled its beds.

The drama of trying to limit the damage from disease and to delay death often came down, in reality, to following up on details. Weekends and holidays the on-call intern received a list of requests for assistance from the other interns on the team who described in detail the care their patients needed. "If possible" was written beside much of what should be done on the Team C list. We all recognized that everything could not be done; Team C had a reputation as one of the rotations that could "hurt interns the worst." (The phrase bred of fatigue belied the fact that the patients were the ones who were hurt.) The team was too large and too spread out through the hospital.

The sickest children had to be taken care of first.

Joy was one. She had not even had a first birthday when she lay dying in the intensive care unit. She had been hooked to the respirator for weeks, unable to breathe on her own, growing progressively worse with pneumocystis pneumonia. Critically ill, tortured by the infections her damaged immune system could not fight, unresponsive to antibiotics, she clearly seemed to be dying.

Pneumonia, which in someone without AIDS normally involves only a part of the lungs, had spared none of Joy's. The X ray of her lungs should have been filled with black, portraying healthy breathing space; Joy's was completely covered by the white of pneumonia. The medical team debated whether to prolong her painful life and postpone her inevitable death by continuing to keep her on the respirator — tubes feeding her, and plastic going into her throat, her windpipe, her tiny urethral opening, her veins, and arteries — or whether to begin to disconnect the tubes and try to help her die as peacefully as possible. Together with her mother, the decision was made: a "DNR" (do not resuscitate) order was written in her chart. The DNR order meant that if her breathing stopped as everyone expected when the respirator was gradually disconnected, the ventilator would not be reconnected. But she would be fed. She would be given everything to make her comfortable.

Joy gave every indication of being dependent on the respirator to breathe. The team of doctors, nurses, and respiratory therapists who worked with her around the clock began to disconnect it in order not to protract what seemed inevitable. Although the medical team and Joy's family stopped fighting her illness, Joy fought to survive any way she could. Days later, off the ventilator and out of the intensive care unit, she lay in her crib on a regular hospital floor in a Team C bed. It still took no more than a glance into her room to see how sick she was. At eight months old, she looked the size of a baby only a quarter her age. Her skin clung tightly to her bones. She had an oxygen mask over her face, and her chest was still going up and down at twice the normal rate as she gasped for air. She was connected to both cardiac and respiratory monitors to sound the alarms if the enormous efforts that her little body was making ceased to be enough. She was a jungle of wires monitoring her heart and lungs, and tubes for providing her with food, fluids, and medicines.

The first night after Joy was transferred out of the intensive care unit to the regular floor, we worried that Joy would worsen hourly and die. Joy continued living on the margin, her lungs always critically close to failing completely, but nonetheless breathing on her own. Her mother, Esper, stood constant vigil by her bed. Joy's father had become infected with HIV through intravenous drug use, and Esper had become infected through sexual relations with him. Joy had become infected in the womb.

As Esper stood watch over Joy, I asked her whether she had taken the time to get medical care for herself to help her avoid contracting the pneumocystis pneumonia that riddled Joy's lungs. I wondered about Esper's feelings as she saw her daughter suffer with HIV, which plagued them both. But if in fact Esper worried about her own fate, her fears were closely guarded. All her questions were about Joy. Each time someone came into the room, she asked their opinion: "Will Joy ever make it home? Even for a couple days?"

As Joy's health gradually improved, we all began to hope Joy might make it home. Unable to talk, Joy gave every other indication of struggling to stay alive. We thought if she had a respiratory arrest now, resuscitation might be able to pull her through in good enough condition that she could eventually go home. After discussions with her mother, Joy's DNR came off the books.

Joy's mother and grandmother kept a vigil at her bedside until she was ready to go home. After Joy's discharge, I would sometimes see Esper walking through the hospital lobby on her way to Joy's checkups. Esper was always wheeling a large oxygen tank in one hand, carrying Joy in the other, and repeatedly disentangling the tube in between.

We know so little about why the health of some children with AIDS holds out much longer than others'. At seven years of age Marguerita had stayed healthy for much longer than Joy. Marguerita's and my friendship grew during her hospitalizations. When I first helped care for her pneumonia and pancreatitis, we planned her birthday party and how to get her home in time for it. She made it home belatedly.

Each time I heard she was back in the hospital, I was scared it might be the last time. The question was never whether she would come back to the hospital; it was whether she would leave. Throughout my internship, I visited her in the hospital even when she was not my patient. She baked Rice Krispies cookies in the kitchen and brought them to me with pride. We sat together in the lobby and listened to guest rap bands.

We spent time together when she began to grow discouraged. She did not want to talk about her feelings as she grew sadder and more fearful, but she did want us to sit on her hospital bed and make artwork with yarn together. I went into another room to listen to Marguerita's mother when I knew she needed to cry. Marguerita did not want her mother's or anyone else's tears near her room. I knew my own eyes would fill up. The baffling standards of professional distance left a porous barricade.

Caring at the same time for children with both AIDS and aplastic anemia was haunting. Both groups of children are at risk of dying from infection because of an immune system that has shut down. Aplastic anemia is a rare disease that wipes out most of the blood cells and leaves patients as vulnerable to infection as those who have AIDS. But the contrast between society's treatment of children with aplastic anemia and those with AIDS is dramatic. Children with aplastic anemia have a better chance of survival, yet their condition is treated as more tragic. While some children with aplastic anemia become the object of community fund-raising drives to pay for their medical treatment, some children with AIDS become the object of community efforts to have them forced out of local schools and even towns.

Katrina ran energetically around her crib, loudly and happily gurgling to her attentive parents. At fourteen months of age, with beautiful black curls falling onto her full shoulders, long eyelashes shading her big brown eyes, her only discomfort was hunger from an overnight fast ordered by the lung specialist. Her face filled with smiles, her room filled with her coos, she was unaware of anyone's anguish.

A recent blood test had shown that she had antibodies to HIV, but the meaning of that finding is ambiguous in children her age. The test could indicate that she was truly infected with HIV or that she had passively received her mother's antibodies but had not become infected. I wanted so badly for Katrina not to be infected; I could only imagine how desperately her parents must have wanted the same thing. Looking at her I saw no overt signs of illness. As I began her physical exam, my face must have become expressionless. Liver enlarged. Spleen enlarged. Lymph nodes palpable behind her ears, in her neck, beside her clavicles, in her groin. No mistaking it. I could not help but wonder how many strangers, not knowing her HIV-status, would reach out instinctively to her, but knowing it, would shy away.

The morning Katrina came to the hospital was the same

morning that her mother, Mina, found out she had tested positive for HIV herself. Mina had gotten tested as soon as she learned Katrina was infected. After Katrina's stepfather translated the news for Mina, he promised repeatedly to stay with her and Katrina throughout the course of their illnesses, however the illnesses ended. No one could give them a greater gift.

Katrina's biological father had already died of AIDS. He had acquired it through intravenous drug use. Neither her mother nor her stepfather had ever used drugs. Like Esper, Katrina's mother became infected through sexual contact with her father.

Discrimination against those with AIDS has its own hierarchy. Katrina, the "innocent child," received far more sympathy than her mother. If grieving for her daughter's illness and her own was not enough, Katrina's mother had to live with an unbearable burden of guilt. Any parent whose child is seriously ill searches for an answer to what could have been done differently to prevent the disease. Self-recrimination is magnified when there is any suggestion that the child's sickness could have been avoided. On top of her own doubts, Katrina's mother — who did not even know she was infected when she gave birth to Katrina — had to face social recriminations.

Using how people became sick as grounds for prejudice is not new with AIDS. Syphilis was originally seen as a disease that affected only those who had had extramarital sexual relations. That belief changed when people began to realize that children were also becoming infected, and the public started focusing on the notion of the innocence and guilt of those infected. In a debate over standards requiring physicians to report cases of syphilis to the health department, Dr. James Walsh was only one of many who argued, "We surely cannot report the innocent as well as the guilty" (Walsh 1911). Although the words *innocent* and *guilty* are not openly used in HIV policy debates, the power of the prejudice can be seen in the difference between public treatment of the child who is congenitally infected or the adult who is infected by a blood transfusion and the adult who is infected sexually or through intravenous drug use. Today, most of us reading the nineteenth-century satire *Erewhon,* in which people are punished for being sick, would call such treatment implausible. The form of trial may be slightly more subtle today, but the punishment is just as protracted.

Katrina, who had had a chronic cough for months, came to the hospital to have a bronchoscopy performed. The pulmonologists wanted to look for evidence of pneumocystis pneumonia, the same infection that had almost killed Joy. During a bronchoscopy, a long, black, flexible rubber tube is passed down through the throat into the lungs. The tube contains a fiberoptic scope to magnify what is seen, a small pair of scissors for taking samples, and a hose for cleaning the path.

As they waited to hear how the bronchoscopy had gone, Katrina's mother and stepfather sat anxiously gazing out the window. Katrina lay next to them in a tent filled with mist to soothe her throat, sore from the passage of the large bronchoscopy tube.

"Can I hold her now?" Mina asked immediately when she saw me.

"Absolutely." She instantly lifted Katrina from her tent and held her tightly, terrified for Katrina, for her own future, and for that of her three other children.

Researchers estimate that in Africa alone 3.7 million children may be orphaned by AIDS by 1995. There will be many more worldwide. Mina's three uninfected children might join that total. Katrina's stepfather slipped one hand into Mina's and the other around Katrina.

Later that day, the hospital social worker, hardened by hearing too many sad stories for too many years, came back to the ward. Her eyes filled as she held back the tears. Katrina's mother and stepfather had just found out that the public housing authority had given away the apartment they had been desperately seeking. Their turn had come, but they had been unable to make their appointment since Katrina needed them at the hospital.

By the time I had taken care of the children who urgently needed to be seen on Team C on Saturday, it was two in the afternoon. Only then was there a chance to begin taking care of the many details that make a difference in the lives of patients who are not critically ill: changing intravenous medications to oral ones so children can go home, changing feeding regimens, reporting test results to families, and seeing stable patients.

It was two in the morning before all the patients had been seen and test results checked. Then it was time for paperwork. There was a choice, a little like choosing between lima beans and brussels sprouts if you are two years old and hate green vegetables. I could stay up and do the paperwork in the middle of the night or I could stay late the next day.

The next day, a long line of hospital personnel snaked through the lobby for their annual influenza vaccine: doctors, nurses, lab technicians, maintenance personnel, people who empty bed pans, and people who empty the trash. At least the vaccines were available to everyone. I got in line without thinking and then began to worry. In the past, the swine flu shot had been associated with Guillain-Barré syndrome. Normally, I would not have worried. Guillain-Barré is rare, and whether it is truly a complication of flu vaccines is still debated. But Guillain-Barré can be a life-threatening illness, and I had had it once already. Did I have a greater chance of its recurrence than someone who had never had it before?

As I stood in line, memories of having Guillain-Barré during the second year of medical school came back. Suddenly unable to sit upright in the library, recognizing that something was seriously wrong, I had gone to the university health services where I explained, "I feel pretty awful. I don't think I can sit until it's my turn to see the doctor. Is there someplace I can lie down?"

The receptionist let me lie down on a couch. When the doctor saw me there, he made up his mind before he examined me.

"Are things going badly? Sometimes medical school can be tough . . ."

I tried to explain that I loved medical school. Yes, things were going badly, but only because I could neither stand nor sit for any length of time. The physician did not even examine me. He explained how distressing medical school could be and offered to drive me home. I declined his offer and called my family, recognizing that I was too sick to spend the night alone in my apartment.

Early the next morning, I went in to another of the university health services offices. I had realized my symptoms were classic for severe orthostatic hypotension, when blood pressure falls when sitting or standing and not enough blood reaches the brain.

"Would you please check my blood pressure when I'm standing too?" I asked the triage nurse. As she checked my blood pressure, I sat with my legs curled under me to keep from fainting. "I think I may have orthostatic hypotension."

She scowled and, uninterested in taking suggestions from a patient, did not even respond.

The second physician measured my blood pressure while I was sitting. It was too low. While I was standing, he could not even get a reading. He called an ambulance.

Typically, Guillain-Barré syndrome involves an ascending paralysis of the muscles. First, often the feet cannot move; then the legs and the arms. Eventually, in its life-threatening form, the chest muscles are unable to move air in and out of the lungs. Guillain-Barré is a disease of the nervous system and can attack any part of it; in my case it hit the autonomic nervous system, the part that controls blood pressure. It takes weeks and months for the nervous system to heal.

When it was my turn in line for the influenza vaccine, I asked, "Do you advise those who have had Guillain-Barré before to get the flu shot?"

"I don't know," the physician in charge replied honestly. Not enough patients had been studied to know. *We don't know* is the truthful answer to the majority of questions in medicine. I stepped out of line and waited to ask other physicians for their recommendation. Following the advice of several physicians, I did not get the flu shot that year.

Three weeks later, I was home with influenza and a 104-degree fever. My losses were piling up even as I followed medical recommendations: "The risks of the flu shot outweigh the benefits in your case"; "The benefits of surgery outweigh the risks in your case." Perhaps I just lost the gamble both times. Perhaps the odds were actually the reverse of what anyone had known. Research shows that physicians often do a poor job at estimating the risks and benefits of treatment of well-studied diseases. They do even less well when estimating the effect of treating uncommon diseases or conditions that have not been well studied.

After three days of high fever, my temperature finally dropped to 101 degrees. Having convinced myself that I was no longer contagious, I telephoned the senior resident in charge of my team and talked to her about whether to go to work or to wait one more day.

I was falling into a common trap. Jim, one of the brightest and most compassionate physicians I know, fell into the same trap. Worrying about his colleagues, Jim went to work sick in spite of a fever, sore throat, cough, and muscle pains. He was trained to think of the other doctors and to accept a residency system that had no room for doctors in training to get infectious diseases. He reasoned that his colleagues were overworked as it was; he could not ask them to see his patients too.

He described to me the care he had given while sick. He had seen a patient who needed a urinary catheter placed. To limit the pain she would have due to the tube being passed through her narrowed urethra, he went in search of a small catheter. To find one, he had gone into a bone marrow transplant unit, where the patients with no immunity could have been endangered by his illness.

"Couldn't someone else have picked up the catheter?"

"The urologist would've hit the roof if I had told him I didn't want to get the catheter just because I had a sore throat and fever," he explained.

What was I doing even asking about coming in to work, and what was Jim doing staying at work? We were both following common practice. The work ethic among inpatient physicians — go to work as long as you can stand up — is clearly doctor-, not patient-centered. The justification is almost always presented in terms of the burden other physicians would have to bear if the sick doctor were not to show up for work.

The dialogue rarely mentions the patients except in a perfunctory way and certainly does not deal with the question from their perspective. Do patients really want to be seen by a sick doctor? Is the doctor feeling well enough to listen carefully? Is the sick doctor really thinking clearly enough to provide quality care? At the most basic level, is the patient going to get sick if the doctor has an infectious illness and is in close contact?

With permission from the resident, I stayed home the day my fever dropped to 101 degrees, but wondered whether I was being a wimp. I seemed to have largely recovered from the flu until dinnertime, when I could tell I was becoming incoherent. I assumed the incoherence was due to extreme exhaustion and went to bed hoping to be lucid by morning.

At two in the morning, I woke up feeling like I was burning up. As sweat poured off my brow, I coughed constantly, unable to stop even to speak three words with Tim about what to do. He talked; I nodded. Temperature of 105 degrees, violent shaking chills, cough bringing up pus — it was textbook post-influenza pneumococcal pneumonia.

Tim lay in bed and I sat coughing and choking out monosyllables as we discussed whether to go to the emergency room immediately or wait until morning. Images battled each other in my mind. Janis, a fifty-year-old woman I had taken care of when she was comatose in the intensive care unit, had had pneumococcal pneumonia for only twenty-four hours before she came in to see a doctor. By that time it was too late to arrest the tragic process. Within hours, she could no longer breathe for herself. The infection spread to her kidneys and shut them down. She went into fulminant liver failure. She died from a treatable but deadly disease. The twenty-four-hour delay had made the difference between life and death.

Then there was the devil's advocate, who repeated the medical school maxim: students worry too much. Most young and middle-aged adults do fine when they get treatment for bacterial pneumonia within a couple days. I did not want to disturb a lot of people unnecessarily that night. To go to the hospital would mean waking Ben and someone to care for him in the middle of the night. I could not even be certain I had pneumonia until the exam was conducted.

Tim was soothing, bringing cool washcloths. He dealt

with his own fears through well-practiced denial as he nursed me. In the morning he woke up and asked, "Do you want to go to work, Jody?"

Wanting desperately to be well enough to work, hopelessly discouraged at facing another significant illness, I slipped into futile sarcasm. "No, thanks. What do you think about driving me to the emergency room for a little diagnosis?"

We went to Sinai Hospital again. Either because Tim worked there or because we were both doctors, the emergency room staff offered us special treatment.

"If you'd like, we'll just have the attending see you. You don't have to be examined by an intern or resident."

"That's okay. The intern can evaluate me first if he wants." I was coughing too much to try and explain that I was an intern and understood how tightly interwoven training programs and patient care were.

The intern spent most of his time looking in my ears with an otoscope. When he walked out, finding nothing wrong, I whispered to Tim that he had forgotten to listen to the front of my chest, the only place where the right middle lobe of the lung can be heard, and a common site for pneumonia. The horrible hacking cough would have clued the intern in if he had had more experience. In part out of misplaced politeness and in part out of a real recognition that the quality of my care might depend on the intern's goodwill, I was careful about pointing out his omission to him. In our current health care system, even for a doctor it is hard and can be risky to be a forceful advocate for oneself.

One of the strengths of teaching hospitals is that several doctors at different levels of training see each patient. The checks and balances make mistakes and omissions in care less likely.

The attending came and listened to my lungs. He immediately found the pneumonia and requested an X ray, which rapidly confirmed the diagnosis.

"Do you want to stay at Sinai to be treated?" he inquired.

"Do I have a choice?"

The attending explained that given that I was a doctor being cared for by another doctor, Tim, he would feel comfortable treating me at home. "I trust you'd know if you needed to come back into the hospital," he half-stated and half-asked.

"I've spent enough time in hospitals lately. If there's a choice, I'd rather go home."

I couldn't help but think that I was fortunate to have that choice. Billie had a harder time getting home. At fourteen, she had already been in and out of the hospital four times that year with a cough from her cystic fibrosis, which was worsening and signaling probable new infections. She was tired of the hospital. For her, the painful search to place a new intravenous line in her scarred veins each night was almost a diversion from the silence of dealing with the impending death of another patient with cystic fibrosis on the floor, a patient she had known all her life, and who months before had been in the same condition as Billie. Billie knew she was not likely to live a normal life span. It was impossible for her not to know that was true when she watched other teenagers, barely older than she, die from their cystic fibrosis, others whose illness had progressed similarly to hers. She wanted to spend as much time as she could outside the hospital. She knew she needed antibiotics, but she wanted to have them at home instead of in the hospital, either in a spray or an intravenous form that she would have to have hooked up only once a day. But despite the availability of alternatives, the medical team prescribed medications that required her hospitalization.

It was better to be at home than in the hospital as a patient but it was still bad.

I wish it had been like the movies of the 1950s, in which the young woman goes home ready to bear any affliction, always cheery despite the most dire predictions. Between bandages and cooling baths for her fever, she gingerly cooks tenderloin for her children. But I was depressed and feeling like I had lost the match.

When I called the chief resident to let her know what was wrong, Renee's first words were, "I'm so sorry to hear that." Her second sentence followed swiftly: "When will you be able to come back?"

Her words were a reflection not on her or the hospital but on the residency system. One of the engines the hospital depended on was its residents, each working eighty, ninety, one hundred hours a week year-round. Not only did the residency system efficiently exploit a tamed labor force, but it also ran so tightly that it provided little flexibility for foreseeable problems. While any individual's illness was unpredictable, it was readily foreseeable that each year some of the dozens of residents would need to take leave for their own illnesses or to care for sick family members or newborns.

Mark rotated out of the emergency room to cover my place on the ward service while I was home with pneumonia. When I came back after three weeks at home, I took Mark's place in the emergency room.

By noon on my first day back, I had to sit down each time I took a patient's history. By three, I was watching the clock to see if I would make it until five. The last patient I saw that first day was a child who needed blood drawn. When I went to throw out the needle I had used to draw his blood, I stuck myself.

Like many hospitals, Children's Hospital had developed procedures to help prevent the spread of blood-borne diseases and, when not prevented, to help treat them. Every needle stick had to be reported to the employee health office.

The next morning, the employee health nurse asked me to come to her office in the catacombs of the hospital to fill out a report regarding the needle stick. She advised me to ask permission of the patient's parents to test their child's, John's, blood. I had asked for such permission a number of times on behalf of other physicians, nurses, and cleaning staff who had been exposed to the blood of one of my patients. It was routine.

After seeing the employee health nurse, I returned to the emergency room to see patients who had returned from radiology. When I finished taking care of them, I went to speak with John's mother. As I walked to the elevator, I felt faint; I thought about getting a quick drink, if not lunch. But I knew John and his mother were waiting for me; I remembered what it was like to wait to be discharged and I did not want to make them linger until after my lunch. My beeper went off to remind me that they were waiting. As I went up in the elevator, I thought I would be able to take care of everything quickly and then get something to eat and drink.

As I hurried into John's room, everything started to look hazy, and I realized I was about to faint. I had had low blood pressure long enough to know what that felt like. I squatted next to John's mother to talk to her. Bending my legs returned some of the blood to my head and things looked clear and sharp again.

John's mother politely said, "Oh, please sit down."

"No, that's all right. I'm fine."

"Really, please sit down. Make yourself comfortable."

I went to get a chair because I was clearly making her worry by my squatting next to her. As I got up to get the chair, everything started to blur again. I looked outside and could not see a chair, so I came back to squat next to her. Things cleared as soon as I was sitting on the ground, but she stood up from her chair and said, "Please take mine."

I stood up and said, "No, really, sit down, I'll just go find a chair." Again, as soon as I got up, everything became hazy. That time when I left for the chair, I did not come back.

The next thing I remember, someone was coming over to me. "What's going on here?" she asked rapidly.

"She's having a seizure." More and more people started coming over.

"She's getting cyanotic." Blue in the face. Urgent now. "Get a tongue blade."

Another voice, "No, get an oral airway." Increasingly urgent. A code was called.

I thought to myself, "No, just turn her on her side." I had been through this before as a physician, but now my role had changed. As I watched everyone gather around and conduct the emergency procedures they had been trained to do so well, I felt part of the routine. Enough a part of it to think about what the right approach was to someone who was seizing: turn her on her side to prevent aspiration — as long as she is breathing well enough on her own . . .

Then I recognized that I was on the wrong side. More and more people kept gathering around, and the voices kept talking about me.

"She can't move her right side."

I thought, I haven't tried.

"Get an IV."

"Load her on Dilantin."

Then someone began talking to me. "Squeeze both hands." I was still looking around trying to absorb it all, my attention staccato. Someone said, "Squeeze your right hand." My right arm hurt from the IV placement and Dilantin flowing in. "Your left hand."

"Are you on any meds?"

"Yes, Tegretol. I was about to take my midday dose."

"Any others?"

"No."

"She's dysarthric," they said to each other, referring to an apparent inability to articulate my words, but my voice sounded normal to me. (Later, the physician who had found me seizing would describe my speech as not slurring but choppy.) A voice, which turned out to be a fellow intern's, shouted from the nursing station, "We'll call your husband. What's his number?"

"We're going to take you to the Brigham and Women's Hospital," someone explained. The next-door hospital for adults and newborns was connected by an indoor tunnel.

A resident and Kit, an attending anesthesiologist who had come when the code was called, wheeled me over on a stretcher. Before leaving me in the hands of the Brigham emergency department doctors, Kit asked at the door, "Is there anyone special at Children's you want me to ask to come over?"

"No, that's okay. My husband's coming. Thanks so much for all your help."

When Kit asked if I wanted him to send someone over, it made me realize that while I was thinking I'm doing okay, I've felt much worse, I'm just a little worried, I must have looked sick, scared, alone, and physically at risk. Kit wrote Tim's name and phone number on the sheet beneath me — just to make sure the emergency room physicians knew how to find him if I began to seize again.

Then I was alone. An oxygen mask covered my nose and mouth. As Dilantin dripped in through the intravenous line in my arm, I tried to concentrate on piecing together what had happened.

Was the intravenous Dilantin necessary to stop the seizure

activity, or had it been given to me reflexively by the physicians who first discovered me on the floor? If emergency medical treatment had been necessary to stop the seizure and prevent status epilepticus, then it would be far more dangerous to return overseas to remote areas. The fact that seizures and attempts to avoid them would continue to affect my daily life in the United States had not yet dawned on me; I was still concentrating on how seizures would affect long-held dreams.

Tomas Garcia walked in and introduced himself as the emergency room attending. There was a calm caring in his voice and face, a reassuring absence of pressure, panic, or signal of tragedy. I told him and the neurology resident the details I could remember, one after the other. Dr. Garcia was certain that the episode was convulsive syncope. The neurology resident was equally convinced it could not be; he argued that convulsive syncope was uncommon. "Unless," as he put it, "you faint in a telephone booth. If you faint and don't fall down, then your brain doesn't get enough oxygen, and you can have convulsive syncope."

Even people who do not have epilepsy, who have never had a seizure before in their life and who may never have one again, can have some of the same muscular movements as seizures when they faint. The medical term is *convulsive syncope.* My hopes of getting off anticonvulsants in time to have a medication-free pregnancy were far greater if I had had convulsive syncope than if I had had another straight seizure. Overseas, the risks associated with fainting would be fewer than those accompanying seizures. At the first sign of lightheadedness, I would be able to move away from the dangers of losing consciousness while cooking over a fire or hiking on a steep trail to reach a refugee camp.

After being discharged, walking through Children's Hospital to get my winter parka, I ran into Chris, a fellow resident.

He stopped me. "How's your arm?" He had put in the intravenous line.

"Fine, thanks," I answered, awkward at the change in our working relationship. "Do you know who found me first?" I nonetheless asked, set on finding out what had happened.

"Cathy. You know? From Ear, Nose, and Throat."

I spoke with Cathy on the phone that night. She had been walking by and had found me unconscious, being held up by a nurse. Dr. Garcia was right. The nurse had been the telephone booth. The memories did not come flooding back, but trickled in over days, completing the picture as slowly as drops would fill a glass with water. I had gone to ask the nurse where there was a place to sit down while talking with John's mother. Then I blacked out. The nurse must have caught me upright.

Cathy went on to describe that then my left arm began to tremble. My left leg began to move next. My back arched. My jaw clenched down.

"Did the seizure stop before they gave me Dilantin?" I asked.

"Yes."

"So I stopped seizing on my own without any medications?" I asked again in different words to make sure. That was the single-most important detail for being able to work again in remote areas.

"Yes."

When the issue of the medical school alumni bulletin came, there was a photo essay about what it means to be a patient: "Images of Illness: The Person Behind the Patient." One picture showed a patient with all his bottles of medicine. Another picture showed a patient lying on a gurney on his way into surgery with his hair net on. A third picture showed the same patient in the operating room, cut open. But time spent as the subject of a code reminded me that these were pictures of patients, not pictures from the patient's point of view, as they were supposed to be. They presented sights the patients never see. He sees the basket of medicine grow. He sees the ceiling of the halls on the way to surgery through a drug-induced fog. When he sees the code, he sees the doctors' faces and hands, not his own. He feels his own presence but never sees it. If they had wanted to show the patient's view, the pictures should have been taken from home plate, not from the pitcher's mound.

CHAPTER EIGHT

Chiapas, Mexico

The opposite of love, I have learned, is
not hate but indifference.

—*Elie Wiesel*

IN AUGUST, when I had recovered from neurosurgery
enough to sit up and write but not enough to walk and be
active, I longed for a meaningful way to spend time. I had been
asked to be a member of the board of directors of Partners in
Health and to help provide support to projects in Central
America. Partners in Health is a public charity, which grew out
of work in rural Haiti and whose goal is "to improve the health
of underserved communities and to foster active community
involvement in the planning and implementation of efforts to
maintain health and overcome illness."

   For several years, study and research had repeatedly taken
me to Mexico and Guatemala. Working with Partners in
Health at last gave me the opportunity to provide more meaningful support to colleagues in Mexico than documenting the
problems did. Health conditions in Guatemala were among the
worst in the hemisphere; Guatemala had the highest age-
adjusted death rate of all thirty-one Latin American countries
and territories for which the World Health Organization had
information. Two out of three children under five suffered

some degree of malnutrition and more than one in ten infants died before his or her first birthday. Few resources were available to combat the conditions; the combined public and private spending on health care was only $23 per capita. Military dictatorships and political repression, including the killing and disappearance of over one hundred thousand citizens during two decades, had led tens of thousands of Guatemalans to go into exile in southern Mexico in the early 1980s. After fleeing through the mountains without food, the refugees arrived in Mexico in even worse health than when they had left Guatemala. Among children, the annual death rate reached the equivalent of nearly 11 percent.

On behalf of Partners in Health I wrote letters to health care projects that served Guatemalan refugees, inviting applications for funds. Guatemalan and Mexican colleagues responded with a proposal to train health care workers. Together we scheduled a project site visit for April.

By April, the passage of time and the experience of living daily with the risk of seizures had worn down to a manageable size any fear I had of traveling to remote regions. I could still remember sitting up at night thinking sadly about coding Mark for status epilepticus, but I was no longer sleepless. I knew that status epilepticus in a foreign village or refugee camp without health care could mean death or a life so damaged and disabled as to be unrecognizable. But the last seizure, in February, had been strangely reassuring. Like the overwhelming majority of seizures, it had stopped on its own. Conversations with health care workers in rural Mexico had forewarned me that a straightforward seizure while traveling still carried the risk of broken teeth from well-meant but ill-advised attempts to force a spoon between my teeth, of injections with contaminated needles if an attempt was made to give medication, or of witnesses believing I was possessed.

Still frightened, but yearning to resume work in Mexico and Guatemala, I packed my bags the Friday night that my vacation began and left Saturday morning for a trip that had been conceived in a dream and carried out, as many dreams are, in stolen time. The night before I left Cambridge, Ben and I took out his bubbles to play.

By the middle of the next day, my flight landed in Mexico City. The mountains surrounding the city were made invisible by pollution, among the worst in the world. A connecting flight landed in Tuxtla, in the south of Mexico, where the smoke from fires burning the cropland clear made the sky as impenetrable as that surrounding Mexico City.

My colleagues came to get me in Tuxtla. In the back streets leading to the market, the overpowering smell of guava permeated a hundred-foot radius. From a distance, the watermelon looked picture-perfect, bright red perspiring pieces filled with sharp black seeds, until you walked by. Then half the seeds flew away. In the central square, hundreds of people were spending the weekend day with their children. In the far corner, a grandfather blew bubbles for his toddler.

We left Tuxtla after lunch. By night, the landscape was scattered with as many small flames as the sky was with stars. We drove to San Cristóbal de las Casas, a town in the mountains. The next day, we prepared to leave San Cristóbal de las Casas and drive for the Guatemalan refugee camps. Our departure for the refugee camps was delayed by the need for truck repairs. The truck's battery was held in place by a string lasso. The oil line was fixed with a rubber gasket we had cut in the dark the night before from the inside of the truck's roof.

While the truck was being repaired, I read a health bulletin about epilepsy printed for the refugee health workers. It described in writing what I had been warned about over the phone. As in the United States, misconceptions about seizures were widespread. Some people still believed that seizures were caused by witchcraft or by the devil. The bulletin showed a picture of a whole village running with machetes in hand after a person who had had a seizure. The bulletin explained that seizures were not caused by the devil and went on to recommend purportedly modern treatments. Even some of these recommendations, however, had long since proved hazardous.

After the truck's oil line was fixed, three health care workers, two grandmothers, their granddaughter Marta, who had been in the hospital, and I set off for one of the refugee camps. Shivering in the morning mountain air, I rolled up the front window only to find that the breeze remained just as strong. There was a four-inch gaping opening between the cab and the bed of the truck. José informed me calmly that the gap was old and not widening. Marta's small six-year-old hand bridged the gap. She sat on her grandmother's lap and leaned over to pat my head.

The land on either side of the road into the refugee camps had changed dramatically over the years. Originally cut through dense rain forest famous for its beauty and its birds, the road now ran between barren hillsides. Coming back year after year, watching the rain forest change to mud slides, was like watching a video on fast-forward. The irreversible loss of natural resources could have been prevented. Without stoves, the refugees depended on the trees for wood for cooking. They had traveled farther and farther from their villages to chop down trees each year. Needing regularly to clear new land for farming, without the equipment and supplies that would have made less land-intensive methods of farming feasible, they had slashed and burned the remaining woods.

After twelve hours driving on sand and gravel, we arrived at the end of the resurfaced dirt road. It stopped as suddenly as the funding to the refugee camps had. Our speed fell from

twenty miles an hour to five as we encountered foot-high
mounds and deeper ditches spaced no farther apart than the
jeep's wheels. Our clothes were coated with dried dirt from
the road. Everyone's hair was colored a reddish brown.

After several more hours of driving, we came to the end
of the dirt road, and it was time to walk the rest of the way to
the camp, one of the closest ones. Other camps were a several
days' walk away.

As we walked through burning fields, my cough rapidly
worsened. I had begun to cough in the brief stopover in
Mexico City's polluted skies. The coughing had increased
while driving out of Tuxtla on roads shouldered by burning
fields and while driving into the camps on the dirt roads.
Now in the camps, hours from any clinic or hospital, my
breathing became shallower and shallower as the bronchi that
led from my windpipe to lungs reacted in spasms to the dust
and soot, which now coated them. Like straws, which are
easy to sip through when round but difficult when bitten flat,
my bronchi let little air pass. Talking or making any sound
other than gasping for air became rapidly impossible.

All we had with us for reactive airway disease was an
inhaler of medication, which a Mexican colleague had suggested we buy when the cough was still mild. I kept repeating
the inhaled dose until I could breathe, although with each
dose my heart sped faster, a serious side effect of frequent
use. Since I had no known reactive airway disease or asthma, I
had not expected the marked worsening of the cough over
hours and minutes.

But now for the first time, it was clear that I had developed reactive airway disease after pneumococcal pneumonia.
We sat down on the stripped hillside and looked at the fires
coming from the small surrounding fields.

*   *   *

At dusk we arrived at Rahel's home in the camp. Two men were going from hut to hut selling mangoes and tomatoes. Rahel was cooking dinner over hot coals at one end of her home as her children encircled her, vying for attention and for an early tortilla. Rahel kept urging her cousin, Juliana, who had just given birth to her second child, to sit on the mud floor and rest. Their husbands and unmarried brothers sat in a circle at the other end of the hut on child-size three-legged wooden stools designed to be stable on the cracked mud floor. As a doctor, I was invited to eat with the men. On other days, after my asthma was better, I would decline and eat with the women, but not on that first night, as the women sat together around the smoking ashes of the fire.

Families were at once divided and united by their flight from Guatemala. Families that for generations had lived together in one small village were strewn across the continent, with brothers in Canada, sisters in the United States, and the uncertain possibility of survivors in Guatemala. Those who escaped together to Mexico often shared the same room.

We slept twelve in Rahel's one-room hut. Plastic sacks emptied of donated food were used to fill the cracks in the wooden walls. Three canvas sacks on the mud floor served as roll-away beds for guests. Boards left over from building the house were laid on the sacks for special guests. As Luis laid out the boards, Angelita, keeping her two tiny toddler's feet together, jumped from one board to the next. The youngest children, those who had known no other life, those who had not known the torture and killing their families fled, played happily with toy cars made out of cans and used batteries. Elena wanted to choose her dress to wear, not the T-shirt her mother had picked out. Like Ben, Luisito wanted to eat his mother's food, not his own. Failing that, he wanted to be allowed to tell his parents where to sit.

The hard-packed mud floor would have been easy to sleep on had it not been for the babies and toddlers crying inside and the dogs and roosters responding outside, like members of an out of tune chorus practicing throughout the night. Rare quiet moments were interrupted by the buzz that preceded the frequent bites of mosquitoes.

The refugees were allowed to farm only a small allotment of communal land — not enough to subsist on — even though their homes were now surrounded by vacant mountainsides. They were forced to leave the camps to find day labor in order to survive. From four-thirty to five-fifteen in the morning, Juliana's brother tried repeatedly to rouse her to cook him breakfast before he had to walk up the road to catch a ride in the back of a pickup to find work. The employers, knowing the opportunities for refugees to work were limited, paid only $1 a day, not enough to subsist on.

By dawn, the village paths began to fill with women carrying tortilla dough and water from the wells.

During my visit to the camps, the village health care workers gathered for a course in which the experienced trained the inexperienced using pictures and practice. Before eating together, we all huddled together to wash with water from a tin cup (there was no running water) since we would be eating with our hands. We lined up at the end of a room filled with kitchen smoke from a wood fire. We each received two ladles of watered-down beans and took them to the long wooden table on which cold tortillas had been placed. The tortillas were not enough to remove the taste of mold from the old beans, but the lunch was what the health care workers could afford, and it filled our stomachs before the afternoon's work. The health care workers were all volunteers in their communities, teaching about clean water, helping build latrines, seeing sick patients in a one-room hut called a clinic, and visiting patients in the middle of the night. Some volunteered for months and then tired. Many had been working for years.

The last long table at which I had sat to discuss international health seemed further removed than the stars and far less luminescent. Researchers around the world had gathered in Europe. Waiters served three-course meals daily. A maître d' chose the wine. The tables at which we ate were covered with crystal and silverware carefully placed on a white tablecloth. The kitchen was as removed and invisible as the people affected by any policies recommended — too far removed.

The richness of the table setting in Mexico was the refugee health care workers who sat at it.

Javier was a student in the course. He had worked in Guatemala organizing into cooperatives farmers who were too poor to make a living alone. According to a U.S. Agency for International Development report, Guatemala had the greatest inequality in land distribution in Latin America. On the smallest plots, farmers could barely subsist. In cooperatives they could afford the equipment and supplies to improve their lives. Javier was kidnapped, tortured, and imprisoned without trial; no charges were brought against him except helping people form cooperatives, teaching people to work together. In the early 1980s, he escaped the secret prison where he was held and left the country along with tens of thousands of Guatemalans who fled to Mexico. More than forty thousand ended up in refugee camps in southern Mexico. Like many others, he traveled on foot across the mountainous border with Mexico. He settled in Chiapas with nothing; the people of Chiapas shared with the fleeing refugees their land, agriculture, language, culture, and poverty. In the refugee camps, the health conditions were initially even worse than they had been in Guatemala. Javier decided to learn to be a village health worker.

Raul had only an elementary school education but he was

training health promoters. He had learned enough to provide basic health care. He organized the program to teach other refugees, and looked for funding — just enough to pay for paper and pens, for refugees to take buses and trucks to attend the courses, and to eat beans and tortillas while they were away from their own camps.

Armando had been a village health worker for more than seven years. While Raul was a born storyteller, Armando had learned silence. He broke that silence only to care for patients and train other refugees to provide health care. His service had begun in rural Guatemala, where few physicians worked and health conditions were poorest. When Armando was becoming a rural health worker, over 70 percent of births in the department of Guatemala were attended by a physician, compared with less than 1 percent of deliveries in some rural areas. For many, the only health care they would receive was from village health care workers unable to read or write, trained by pictures and by trial. They worked out of commitment to their communities. But village health workers, who had been relatively safe in the 1970s, were killed in the early 1980s by right-wing death squads for continuing to do public health work. Eventually Armando and his family fled. Armando's face was scarred by the violence of poverty and discrimination. His life was scarred by the war.

Raul, Armando, and two other trainers provided support to 210 health promoters like Javier, almost all of whom were men. The need for women health care providers was painfully reinforced as women approached me with problems they had had for lengthy periods but had not discussed with male health care workers. Many were embarrassed to talk to or undress in front of a male health promoter from their small village. Many had specific concerns related to their reproductive health.

One woman had lost a pregnancy a month before my visit

and now had fever and lower abdominal pain. I sat in her family's smoke-filled hut trying to persuade her husband to ask her the details of the miscarriage or abortion. Her husband said when she was four months pregnant she went and worked very hard as a cook, and that had caused the miscarriage. I worried that she had not told him the whole story, but there was no way to find out. She lay on her wooden bed, lost in pain, imprisoned by her inability to speak Spanish and my inability to spcak any of the Indian languages. The darkness of the camp was broken only by our one candle. A female health promoter who spoke her language could have unlocked her cell of pain in privacy without the presence of her husband as a translator.

In the health promoters' course, none of the trainers were women. Raul had recognized the importance of women health care providers and had gone house to house in one camp looking for students. Women were interested, but their husbands and fathers often would not allow them to travel to another camp to take a course. One of only four womcn students, Valentina, had to receive permission from her husband to attend the course. She had to travel two days, largely on foot, with her infant on her back and her toddler in her arms. While the men who were students were served breakfast in the morning by the families with whom they stayed, she and the other women woke before dawn to cook for the relatives they visited. Her children stayed with her during the course. She tried to practice giving an injection while bending to the ground carrying the weight of her youngest child. She learned what to do over her toddler's cries and in between breaks for breast-feeding.

I joined the refugee health promoters in their daily work. Three large stones beside the main footpath through the camp marked their medical conference room. The health promoters had meticulously documented month after month each child's weight and height. Following children's growth is one of the best ways to detect occult illnesses as well as malnutrition. We flipped through the children's growth charts until we came to one that showed the ominous signs of a child having suddenly fallen markedly off her growth curve. We immediately set out together to try and find her home.

The child was in her one-room house, with a dusty floor of dried mud and a smoking fire inside. The room echoed with the coughs of children. Her mother sat on the edge of the one bed in the hut — narrow and wooden — her eyes on the floor, her head hanging down and shoulders limp in painful resignation.

"Where is Elena?" we asked.

Elena's comparatively healthy three-year-old bulk slept quietly below a blanket. What shook us was Josephina, her mother.

The story came out a tooth at a time. Josephina had been treated three times for pulmonary tuberculosis. The last time she and her husband had gone to the hospital a physician had accused Josephina's husband of having caused her relapse by not ensuring that Josephina finished the antibiotics prescribed. The doctor went on to say that Josephina's tuberculosis was now resistant to the first-line antibiotics and that she would probably die because the usual treatments were no longer effective. "Besides, what medicines remain are very expensive," he added. Was there anything more devastating left for the physician to say?

Josephina's and my own history of tuberculosis stood in naked contrast. In 1976, after I returned from living in Iran as an exchange student, my doctor had placed a routine test for tuberculosis on my arm. When a huge welt on my arm marked a positive test, he took X rays, which demonstrated a small nodule in my lung. It had been caught too early to even be symptomatic. He started me on antituberculosis drugs, which eradicated the disease. Close follow-up showed no return a decade and a half later. Growing up in middle class America with access to preventive medicine and primary care had meant the disease never took its toll.

Josephina, her whole body trembling with her cough, her limbs and chest as skeletal as a person liberated from a concentration camp, her hopes far more bleak, lay opposite me. She lived far from any hospital. She had tried to seek treatment but had not been able to afford to continue the whole course of antibiotics. Discontinuing antibiotics while she had tuberculosis meant that each subsequent course would be less and less effective.

Although we did not know yet for sure, Elena, her daughter, had probably contracted tuberculosis and was in the early stages. With weight loss, a chronic cough, and exposure to her mother, she had three strikes against the improbable hope of being free of infection. Her infection could have been prevented for less than $1 a day—more money than her family had, but not more money than we could afford to spend as a world community on a life.

We urged Josephina to come with Elena back to the hospital with us the next day so they could both receive treatment.

"They told us there were no more effective treatments," Josephina's husband replied in despair.

"We just looked at the bottle of medication that she was taking, and there are other treatments," we tried to explain.

"But we have no money, and the children barely have enough to eat," her husband said, a fact confirmed by the small amount of thin bean porridge they were eating as they huddled on the floor around the fire. Their last trip to the hospital had cost a month's wages just for transportation, food, and lodging.

"You can get a ride to and from the hospital with us, so there will be no transportation costs," we added.

"But who will pay for the medicines?" He had been through this before and knew there was one barrier after another.

"We will help you pay for the medicines. But you will need to come with Josephina. You know how the hospital works. Someone needs to be with her to get food for her, to cook it and take it to her."

"Who will care for our other children while we're both gone?" Each question arose from the pain of previous hope and disillusion.

"We'll give you time to arrange for someone else in the camp to take care of them." Simple to say but not to do when each family barely had enough food for themselves and when he would not be able to work in the fields or provide money for his children while at the hospital.

"I'll help you find someone," interjected Raul.

"I'll also need someone to take care of our plot of land; without the maize, we'll starve in the months to come." Living on the margin, there was no room to spare.

The arrangements took all night. The packing took only minutes: beans and corn were stuffed into an empty grain sack along with one change of clothes, which was all they had.

A woman who had run through the camp looking for us found us after an hour in Josephina's home.

"Will you please come and see Ana right away?" she asked breathlessly. "She's pregnant and having pains in her stomach. It's too early for the baby to come."

We found Ana in the one-room house that she and her husband shared with her two married brothers, one married sister, and all of their children, in a six-foot-square curtained-

off corner that she and her husband called their own. She lay on
a homemade wooden bed, her pregnant weight cushioned only
by their one wool blanket, sweat pouring from her forehead,
the muscles of her face pulling her eyes closed and her mouth
into a grimace of pain. Raul felt her belly and roughly measured the size of the fetus with his hands. "I think she's only
seven months pregnant," he said. He took a fetal stethoscope, a
glorified name for the hollowed-out piece of wood six inches
long that he placed between his ear and her abdomen. Leaning
against it with half of his weight, he tapped out the fetal heart
rate with his left hand. He was skilled.

Opposite the bed was a dark windowless adobe wall.
There on the dirt floor sat the four traditional birth attendants, who had learned midwifery over many years from the
women who had practiced their trade before them. They had
all come from neighboring villages when they heard the call of
a woman in distress.

Feeling Ana's abdomen, soft from the absence of contractions, Raul did not believe she was in early labor. Hearing the
constancy of her pain, sensing her fever, he nonetheless worried that her illness could be an infection that might threaten
the fetus.

"Will you be able to stay and watch Ana tonight?" he
asked, looking at the wall of traditional birth attendants. He
would be working in another village that night.

For the next hour Raul taught each one in turn how to
listen to the fetal heart rate and how to use the thermometer
to gauge Ana's temperature. They listened to the fetal heart
rate in pairs, one holding the fetal stethoscope, awkwardly at
first, in her right hand and tapping out the heartbeat with her
left. The second counted the beats while watching the second
hand on the watch Raul left behind. Three could not tell
time, but they could tell when the second hand had made a

full sweep. The midwives told the figures to the one member of the family who knew how to write numbers. He wrote the results on a sheet that Raul would be able to see the next morning. If the numbers got too high or too low, a messenger would be sent on foot at night to the neighboring camp, where Raul would be.

When we came back the next morning, Ana's fever was already subsiding. The fetal heart rate was strong. Her pains were diminished. In refugee camps with no doctors, no nurses, no clinics, no hospitals, no obstetricians, and no schools, the health promoters were building a health care system from the ground up.

Many women were not as lucky as Ana. Augusto's mother was one that year. Augusto lay in a hut shared by three families, in a curtained-off four-by-six-foot space he shared with his surrogate parents. At eight months, with a body the size of a one-month-old's, he was too weak even to lift his head. As his surrogate father picked him up, yellow stool the consistency of water shot out of him with the force of a garden hose. Augusto's story and that of his mother were tragically common in impoverished areas of developing countries. His mother had died in labor, joining more than half a million women who die each year worldwide from pregnancy-related complications compounded by inadequate access to health care.

The health of mothers and infants was bound together all the more tightly by the poverty of surrogates. Augusto was adopted by his aunt and uncle, but his aunt had no breast milk, not having recently given birth, and no money for formula. She had been mixing water with flour donated by international aid organizations for adults to feed to Augusto. The flour was an inadequate diet for infants. The water was contaminated with infectious organisms. The bottle sat in the kitchen filled with a stale green liquid in between feedings.

Antonio, also bottle-fed and also suffering from severe diarrhea, was even more malnourished than Augusto. We had visited him in the hospital on the way to the refugee camps. His face was that of an old man's, with the skin covering his bones like plastic wrap. The only thing he could move were his small brown eyes. He had long since stopped sucking and was fed by a tube passed through his nose to his stomach. His father, out of fear or in an attempt to distance himself, no longer held or touched him. But when I sat next to Antonio and stroked his head of hair, red from marasmus, he immediately paid attention. His glazed look turned directly toward me, and he followed me carefully with his hollowed-out eyes.

Before leaving the camp, I was asked to see a twelve-year-old boy, Julio. Chronic illness and malnutrition had left him little taller than a six-year-old. The look in his eyes could have come from a wealthy boy with asthma in New York as easily as from a boy in the camps. The look is the look of air hunger. He was looking straight ahead, concentrating too hard on breathing for his eyes or mind to wander. He had too little air to expend even on moving his neck. Under his T-shirt, his chest was being sucked in deeply beneath his clavicles with every effort to move air into his lungs past the closing bronchi. Julio's strained breathing made a high-pitched whistling sound that was audible without a stethoscope.

Julio's bronchial spasms and wheezing grew worse when he went home to get his father. In his house the kitchen was inside. Julio's father had tried to build a partition to keep the smoke from his son, but with the gaps in the wood, the partition hardly helped. Nor did it ease his burden much to go outside, where the burning of the fields still left smoke as dense as a thick fog.

Julio had been to a doctor once at the hospital. Told that

what he had was incurable, he was sent home without the medication he needed. Asthma is a common disease made more common in the camps by the smoke-filled air. While it is incurable, asthma is readily treatable. Yet from a lack of funds and staff, the village clinic had no medication to treat asthma, even in the event of life-threatening attacks. I gave Julio the inhaler that I had brought with me for my cough. I explained its use to him, his father, and the village health care worker. We went over a dozen times in different words not to give the medicine more than once every four hours unless it was an emergency. The village health care promoter had a watch. We went over how to check Julio's pulse as an indicator of side effects.

I worried about how isolated Julio was, about his need for medicine, about the risk to him if the medicine was used incorrectly. Providing health care in remote areas is not like practicing medicine in the United States, where a follow-up appointment for the child can be made readily and where there are doctors nearby if the child gets sicker from either the disease or side effects of the treatment. Raul and I discussed at length how to get treatment for asthma into the camps. I wanted to help build for Julio the health care services everyone deserves, but I needed to do what gave him the best chance of surviving until he had those health care services.

How could a world be just that gave me a so much better chance of surviving airway problems than Julio had, merely because of where we each happened to be born?

On the road back to San Cristóbal de las Casas from the camps, I said good-bye to Raul and Armando; I had no idea that this would be the last time I would see Armando. Months later, the black and white facts would come across the fax in Boston as clearly as the suffering.

The Amnesty International papers read:

URGENT ACTION

"Disappearance" / Fear of Torture / Extrajudicial Execution

Mexico

Armando Mazariegos Paz

Amnesty International is seriously concerned for the physical safety of Armando Mazariegos Paz, whose whereabouts since his abduction remain unknown. According to reports, he was illegally detained at 12:00 P.M., near the train station of the town of Tapachula, in the southern state of Chiapas. According to witnesses, he was forced into an unmarked vehicle by four individuals in civilian clothes who beat him as he tried to resist their assault.

Armando Mazariegos, 35, who is married with two children, is a Guatemalan national who has lived in Tapachula, Chiapas, for the last seven years. He does not have refugee status. He works in the community providing primary health care and is a member of the board of the *Asociacion de Guatemaltecos Refugiados Unidos para Mejorar la Salud (Agrums-association of Guatemalan refugees for improved health care).* He has also given assistance to Guatemalan citizens and refugees.

According to a local radio broadcast (radio XEWM-B) in the town of San Cristóbal de las Casas, his detention was carried out by members of the intelligence service of the Guatemalan army known as G2, who, it is alleged, are active in the border area with Guatemala. Amnesty International has received no further information which would confirm these allegations.

According to reports, in July and August this year, troops of the Guatemalan army have entered Guatemalan refugee camps in Santa Elena Lagartero, Santiago el Vertice and Tziscao inside Mexican territory. There are said to be at least forty thousand Guatemalan refugees living in Mexico.

His abduction was denounced before Mexico's *Secretaria de Gobernacion* (Ministry of the Interior).

Recommended actions: telegrams/telexes/air mail letters.

— Urging immediate clarification of his whereabouts and legal status and that, if in detention, his physical safety be guaranteed, he be allowed access to a lawyer and relatives and immediately released unless charged with a recognizable criminal offense;

— Expressing concern about reports of the possible participation of members of the Guatemalan security forces in the detention of Armando Mazariegos Paz and at the harassment of Guatemalan citizens in Mexican territory and urging Mexican authorities to take up the allegations with appropriate Guatemalan officials.

CHAPTER NINE

Social Problems, Attitudes, and Health

I ARRIVED HOME from Mexico late Sunday night, just in time to start working in the emergency room at Children's Hospital the next day. I must have looked like our 1964 Buick — tired, only running for lack of an alternative.

The contrast with the refugee camps was immediate. Room 14 went up on the emergency room board with a "U" for urgent. A ten-year-old boy named Bill sat rigidly on the Room 14 gurney. His breathing was too restricted for him to talk. His pupils were dilated. His eyes were open wide with fear. He was sitting bolt upright, doing all he could to move air in and out of his lungs.

Treating children in acute respiratory distress is always tricky. They need to be treated quickly so that they can breathe more easily. Treatment often comes before a complete history and physical. The rapid pace that is required can be frightening to both parent and child, and the treatment often involves procedures that are inherently painful, such as inserting needles. Yet swift actions need to be taken in a way that does not intimidate the child. Fear itself can further compromise the child's breathing.

I quickly listened to Bill's chest, learned from his parents that he had a history of asthma and that this attack fit his usual pattern, and then quietly interrupted them and explained, "I just want to get some medicine so we can start making Bill breathe more comfortably, and then we can talk about what he has been going through." Leaving the room, I asked the nearest nurse to start a nebulized treatment of medication — aerosolized medicine that Bill could breathe through a mask.

Bill was clearly in trouble. Lifting his shirt to listen to his lungs, I could see him tugging the front of his chest backward with all his might to within centimeters of his spine in a desperate effort to breathe through contracted airways. He spoke only when directly questioned, and then in whispers to conserve air.

Listening to his chest, I had been able to hear only rare wheezes. Paradoxically, wheezes are rare in both the mildest and most severe asthma attacks. At first, the wheezes are soft and infrequent. As the asthma attack becomes severe, the wheezes grow louder and more pervasive until suddenly, in the most severe attacks, all that is left is eerie silence like in the eye of a storm. Bill's wheezes were rare because he was barely able to breathe.

After using the nebulizer, Bill's wheezes grew into a symphony; the nebulizer would not be enough. I started an intravenous line and admitted Bill to the hospital.

At almost the end of my twelve-to-twelve shift, Kevin, eighteen years old, was wheeled on the run from the ambulance entrance into Room 29, the room in the emergency department reserved for the most urgent medical cases. His arms were covered with bandages where the emergency medical personnel in the ambulance had tried without success to place an intravenous line for medications while the ambulance bounced over the post-winter potholed Boston streets. The ambulance driver gave a two-sentence medical history, and I listened to Kevin's lungs.

"I'm going to start you right away on some medicines to make your breathing easier. Do you have any allergies?"

He shook his head no, and his girlfriend quickly confirmed his answer. He could not force out even a whisper. Within a minute of his arrival, I poured liquid medication into a nebulizer and placed an intravenous line for further treatment. Placing an intravenous line in his veins, pipelines enlarged to feed his muscular physique, was easy in the motionless emergency room.

Once Kevin's breathing eased enough for him to talk, I went back to the emergency room desk to book him a hospital admission bed.

Bruce, a supervising physician in the emergency room, said, "Jody, I have to tell you something about that guy. One of the scariest nights I've ever had in the emergency room was with him. His girlfriend came in semicomatose from too much who knows what drink and drugs. As we were trying to resuscitate her, Kevin and his gang — all the size of linebackers and as doped as hell — started to fight their way into the room."

The contrast between Bruce's experience and mine could not have been more stark. I saw a stoic young man fighting to breathe and his girlfriend standing by his side giving urgently needed medical information. But from the patient's viewpoint the two scenes were consistent and comprehensible. Both involved a young man and a young woman in love fighting for each other's lives. When Bruce had met Kevin, Kevin thought his girlfriend was going to die. Her life was in the hands of people he did not know and had no reason to trust in a world that dished him out a daily diet of discrimination because he was black and poor. He would try anything to get in to see her, to be by her side, to try and protect her. Neither Kevin nor his friends hurt anyone in the emergency room. Yes, he probably was at least drunk but no, his behavior was not incomprehensible to anyone who had walked in his shoes for even a day.

The disparity between what is available to even the poor in the United States in a life-threatening emergency and what is available to the disenfranchised in developing countries could not have been drawn more sharply than by Bill's, Kevin's, and Julio's experiences. Sick with the same condition as Julio, both Bill and Kevin rapidly received the best available treatment. Aerosolized medication was delivered through special equipment that moisturized the air. Simultaneously they received medication through a line placed almost immediately into a vein in their arms. Their heart rates were electronically monitored to alert the team instantly to any serious side effects the medication might be having on their hearts. A team of nurses and physicians came into their rooms frequently to monitor their breathing. As soon as the patients stabilized, there were hospital beds for them with round-the-clock care.

In contrast, Julio had a two-inch handheld dispenser of medication and a father newly trained to take his pulse. If the medication did not work, there was no emergency room. The only round-the-clock care was from a devoted village health worker who had had no training before that day in the treatment of asthma and had no other medications for asthma at his disposal. Even the availability of the one handheld inhaler was a fluke.

The overwhelming majority of international health programs do not provide support for curative care; they fund only public health work. Public health work is essential, but to rely only on public health measures is the equivalent of returning the United States to the eighteenth century — no adequate hospitals, pharmacies, surgery, or medications. To provide only for public health measures is to accept Julio and millions of others dying needlessly from readily treatable conditions.

One after another, patients in the emergency department starkly illuminated the entanglement of social and medical problems. Room 12 was up on the emergency room board. When I went into Room 12, Doug crawled under the chair and fought not to come out. He was a tall, thin seven-year-old. After much reassurance, he was ready to come out, only to go back under the chair when the nurse entered. Finally reassured again, he came out and sat on his mother's lap. He haltingly described to me what had happened.

"I was lying on my tummy . . ."

His mother interrupted, "He used to love to sleep on his stomach."

He continued, "I didn't even hear him come into the room." He paused before crying out, "He put his penis in my bottom."

These frank, painful statements were the only sentences Doug said. The rest of the time he kept saying only "no, no, no, no."

His mother went on: "I was in the bathroom. As soon as I came out, he came to me and told me what Lito had done. I did not know what to do at first. I couldn't believe it. How could this happen?" she asked as if hoping for an answer that would prevent it from ever happening again. "I was afraid but I stood up to Lito. He said, 'What kind of person do you think I am?' I still believed my son and asked Lito to leave, but he wouldn't. He didn't leave the house until a week later when he was arrested for other stuff he'd done."

As we sat alone later in the social worker's office, Doug's mother was finally able to talk about her own fears without worrying that they would further frighten Doug. She spoke haltingly. She explained her fear that her ex-boyfriend would murder her when he found out she had reported his abuse.

"Sometimes I think it would be easier to be dead. Then I wouldn't have to deal with everything."

Yet her love still showed through the cracks in their lives. Her son trusted her and came to her immediately when he was abused. And she responded immediately — steps that do not always happen in cases of abuse. Her love stood out against the backdrop of repeated tragedy. She had been threatened with knives by Lito; she had been sexually abused by him. As a child, she had also been sexually abused. Her older son had been raped when he was out with his friends for a run. As is often the case, sexual and physical abuse was for them an intergenerational tragedy.

To make sure Doug had not contracted a sexually transmitted disease, we would have to take samples from his anus, his urethra, and his throat looking for gonorrhea and chlamydia. I would also need to draw his blood to test for syphilis and HIV. All our efforts to explain that the procedures would be very brief and were to make sure he was not sick and that we would be gentle were to no avail. He was terrified of having the attack repeated. He kicked and screamed when we tried to undress him. Only after forty-five minutes was his mother able to talk him into taking off his shirt and putting on a gown. He repeated again and again, "Why do you want me to? Why do I have to?" His mother kept reassuring him. A half hour passed, and he would not take off his sweatpants. When he finally did, his fear of lying on his stomach was insurmountable.

Unable to concentrate, I paced from one task to another in the emergency room. Acts of nature and acts of God, as terrible as they may be, do not leave the same type of wound as human acts. Doug's and his mother's face were covered with grief at the pain that had been inflicted voluntarily by another human being.

The average wait for patients the next day in the emergency department was several hours, but the triage nurse brought Alicia and her family in right away because of Alicia's strained breathing. She was a beautiful girl with a smile that showed she knew she was loved. She wore five neatly plaited braids. At three and a half, she had already been hospitalized five times for asthma, including once in the intensive care unit immediately after her family had moved into a shelter. Five admissions as a toddler were more than enough to confirm that she had severe asthma. The intensive care unit admission was a further red flag for anyone helping with her care.

Alicia's mother was raising Alicia and her four sisters by herself. The oldest sister was in the eighth grade of a public school where entry was limited to students who scored well on an achievement exam. Her nine-year-old sister, Rena, came into the emergency department with Alicia and their mother. Alicia's mother began describing her vomit from the night before.

"It was bright red."

"Had she been eating anything red? Any red Jell-O, cranberry juice?" I asked, trying to figure out whether the color came from food or blood.

Rena, acting older than her nine years, volunteered to go and get some of the vomit. She had purposely saved a sample. She went alone on the subway to the homeless shelter where they were staying and back to the hospital.

Alicia lay quietly on the gurney talking to herself before we placed a gas mask over her mouth. Unlike most three-and-a-half-year-olds, she was not afraid to sit or lie alone in the hospital emergency room. Her calm betrayed her hard-earned past hospital experience. As I examined Alicia, her mother told me how she and her daughters had come to be homeless.

"It happened when I was·trying to help someone," she began, tears filling her eyes as she recalled the irony. "Another family was evicted. I asked my landlady if I could take them in for a few months while they found a place of their own. I had been living there for six and a half years. She said yes, but then at Christmastime she pretended we had never had the conversation. She said, 'The last ones in have to leave.' I asked if the family could stay just a few weeks longer while the mother was getting on her feet. The landlady said if they did not leave, I would be evicted. They left and I was still evicted."

As she continued, the tears started to stream down her face. "I just don't understand it. I had been living in her house six and a half years. I must have been doing something right. How could she throw us out on the street? I came back and our things were gone. She wouldn't even tell me where the children's clothes were . . . I am so worried about Alicia. Each time she's around someone else who's sick in the shelter, she gets so sick." While we talked, Alicia was already receiving her second nebulizer treatment; her lungs had begun to open up.

Living in a shelter exposed Alicia to a great many of the possible risk factors for future asthma attacks: other children with viruses, smoke, dust and mites, great stress, and often being out in the cold during the day. At her mother's request I wrote a letter to the housing authority about how critical a home was to Alicia's health. It was easy to write; a home is critical to every child's health.

The emergency department has a row of desks and chairs behind a glass wall, which allows doctors and nurses to watch what's going on while conferring privately about patients. This is where residents ask advice from more senior physicians about how to care for patients. This is also where the changing of the guard takes place. Emergency room work is shift work. At the end of each shift, residents sign out and describe and pass on their patients to the next shift.

The area behind the glass was filled when it was time for me to sign out. By the time Jessica, the intern who would be taking over from me, arrived, all the chairs were taken. I offered her mine so she could sit and write notes as I signed out to her. As I kneeled by her side, my head began to spin; I knew I was going down. Quietly but quickly I sat down on the floor. Steve, the emergency department director, immediately asked, "Is something wrong, Jody?"

Knowing my conscious time was limited, I spoke as directly as I could. "I think I'm going to pass out." Worrying about stranding Tim, who was en route to pick me up, I quickly continued, "My husband is coming with the station wagon. . . . He'll be out front. . . . Please let him know." I lay down, hoping that if the dizziness was due to low blood pressure, getting my head below my knees might avert a seizure like the one that had followed the last time I fainted. Unlike in November and in February, this time I knew what was happening and did not feel any sense of panic. I woke up moments later and looked out the door from a stretcher. I realized that I was in Room 29.

Helen, the primary nurse caring for me, had a harsh reputation among medical students. Medical students doing rotations at the end of their fourth year, with little further training, were only weeks away from becoming doctors. But Helen made sure that before they saw any patient, even a patient with a seemingly trivial problem like a cold, they had permission from one of the attending physicians. She wanted to make sure that they did not hurt any of her patients. The medical students knew they needed to be and always were supervised, but making them wait before even beginning to examine a fairly healthy patient seemed punitive to students who had been caring for far sicker patients alone in other rotations.

Helen would not leave my side. Her true colors were clear to her patients. She was as gentle as a lamb and as protective as a lioness. She kept talking to me, reassuring me that I would be fine while others were busy drawing blood and running tests.

The emergency staff is trained for swift action. As soon as I seized, the staff moved ahead of my ability to make any unsolicited requests. Most of my emotions were more human than noble. I was cursing having had another seizure and embarrassed to have had the seizure at work. I was frustrated that as soon as I had had the seizure, they had placed an intravenous line in my arm and loaded my blood stream with high doses of Dilantin, a medication that I now knew from experience would cause low blood pressure problems for days. An ambulance had already been called to ship me to Sinai Hospital, but I did not know why I needed to go to any hospital at all. Most seizures do not require hospitalization.

The dilemma of how to treat seizures is at the same time simple and complex. The basic guidelines are straightforward enough. For people who have had repeated seizures, a recurrence of a seizure that fits the pattern of the person's previous seizures rarely requires either a trip to the emergency room or hospitalization. Whenever an individual has his first seizure or has a seizure that is significantly different from a previous one, that person may require immediate evaluation. Anyone who is having a seizure that does not stop on its own needs emergency treatment as does any person who is having difficulty breathing during a seizure.

Actually following these guidelines, however, is complex.

When a person is found either unconscious or unresponsive, there is no way for a passerby to know what to do; caution dictates getting immediate medical help. But in many cases the person with the seizure is already conscious. One man described having a seizure in a restaurant and quickly regaining consciousness. He and his wife tried in vain to explain that everything was fine. The restaurant owner insisted that they leave by ambulance for liability reasons, costing the family several hundred dollars, and resulting in an unnecessary waste of resources for the community. That one was easy. He could talk. So could his wife.

The physicians at Children's Hospital did not know whether I was just having another seizure, which did not require emergency treatment, or whether I had bled again into my brain.

The ambulance arrived right after Tim. Straps on the gurney brought me barreling back to the world of ceilings, ambulance interiors, and a brief glimpse of the sky. It was finally sinking in that dealing with the risk of seizures would never be over. Failed surgery. Sensitive brain cortex. Whatever the reason. Before, the situation had always been exceptional. Just bled into my brain. Too little anticonvulsant. Recovering from pneumonia. How often do these things happen? Finally, I realized what no one had said. The seizures and their avoidance would always be a presence in my life. Those words are feasible to write now, now that I know more about what they mean. They were unthinkable then.

Dr. Beauregard came to evaluate me in the emergency room at Sinai. She felt it was important to admit me to the hospital and observe me overnight. It was still unclear why I had had another seizure since I had been taking an adequate dose of anticonvulsants regularly. Some people have seizures even on multiple anticonvulsant medications, but my seizures

had seemed fairly responsive to treatment. After one night in
the hospital, she let me go home and prepare to return to
work.

As scared as I had ever been of anything, I was scared the
day I tried to return to work of losing the ability to work,
becoming isolated, and forfeiting friendships and much of what
had meaning in my life. There is a shortcut and a long route
into the emergency room. I took the long path and paused
every step of the way. I stopped inside the glass doorway
terrified of what I would learn.

The reasons to fear employment discrimination were simple.
Discrimination happens time and time again with many types of
disability, and epilepsy is no exception.

The public was asked over a twenty-five-year period, "Do
you think persons with epilepsy should be employed in jobs like
other people?" Benson cited the vast improvement over the
past quarter century, 36 percent more people thought those
with epilepsy should be allowed to work, as wonderful news.
But how low were the numbers to start with that they could
rise so much?

Ignorance forms the foundation for ongoing discrimination. Employers argue that an employee with epilepsy is more
likely to be absent or injured in the workplace. A U.S. Department of Labor study found this was not the case. In fact, studies
have found that the overall absentee rate of employees with
epilepsy is the same as or lower than their coworkers', and
their job performance is the same or better.

Silence conspires to aid and abet ignorance. Like racism,
the discrimination often relies on unspoken but nonetheless
deeply held beliefs that people with epilepsy are less able than
those without. Classes in history, language, and the arts are
often silent about the epilepsy of Alexander the Great, Julius

Caesar, Flaubert, Dostoyevsky, Handel, and many others. With notable exceptions, including past and present U.S. congressmen Coelho and Abercrombie, many contemporary leaders high in the government and academic circles are silent about their own history of seizures because of fear of discrimination. For years on end, they somehow manage never to take their medication in public.

But beyond the impact of ignorance, there is no denying bigotry. A study found that many employers who have hired people with epilepsy and found that these employees are successful remain unwilling to hire others with epilepsy.

In their bulletin, the Epilepsy Foundation of America reports the all too common experiences of people who were about to be offered a job when the employer learned they had epilepsy and then refused to hire them, and of people who were hired and then fired as soon as their employer discovered they had epilepsy.

I heard the same stories over and over at a conference on living with epilepsy held for health care providers, people with epilepsy, and their families. One young man with epilepsy advised others to adopt the following strategy so they would not get fired: "Outperform your peers. Do everything as an overachiever, and they can't fire you. They don't have anything to stand on because you are basically blowing the doors off your peers at whatever you do. You know, be the one that just goes the extra yard all the time." This young man's sadness came out as we listened to the end of conference ceremonial speech. He whispered to me that he had outperformed his peers. He was leading in sales in his company. Then he had a seizure at work. He was told not to come back until he could guarantee that he would never have another one. A physical impossibility.

I was afraid of having damaged friendships with my co-

workers and supervisors, those who had touched me profoundly by the care they had given me, and those who had not
witnessed but had undoubtedly heard of the seizures through
the network of hospital rumors more efficient than the telephone system.

Even if I was allowed to continue work, I was concerned
that people would now see me as "an epileptic" instead of as
Jody, who, among her other attributes, is a person who lives
with seizures. Nor was I alone in these apprehensions. Most of
the people I knew who had had seizures would admit that fact
to no one beyond a close circle of friends and immediate
family.

Knowing the stories of frequent discrimination, I had am-
ple reason to fear it. But my misgivings went beyond that.
Enough prejudice had been internalized before I had seizures
that I could not think very clearly about what would realisti-
cally cause a problem for me in pursuing my work. There was
nothing unique in this. All too often social stigma becomes so
internalized that the victims of discrimination become bigoted
at some basic level themselves: closeted gays who in their
public life work to stamp out homosexuality; African-
Americans who believe being black is base; disabled people
who shrink from their own disability.

During the lunch at the conference on living with epilepsy, Dana, a participant, began to stare. Then her arms began
to move rhythmically, and her face turned uncontrollably to
the right. The movements lasted about sixty seconds. By the
end, a man she had just met was holding her hand, and I had
moved next to her other side to put my arm on her shoulder.
As quickly as the seizure had started, her rigid face softened
into a nervous trained smile filled with embarrassment, and her
blank stare melted into tears.

"I guess I'd better go outside," she said, like a dog running for the door after an accident, stripped of her humanity and her self-confidence.

"You don't have to," I whispered back, stunned at her suggestion.

At that her eyes filled further with tears. Her sense of shame was so ingrained, her humiliation so profound, that even though she was sitting at a table with people who had seizures themselves or who had a family member with seizures she was ready to leave lest she have another.

Later that day, a nurse at the conference told us that she was raised with the knowledge that she had "a seizure disorder." When the term that has been associated with so much discrimination was first applied to her own condition, she was devastated. It had never before occurred to her that she had epilepsy.

As I walked into Children's Hospital's emergency department for the first time since the seizure, I was terrified to face people who had seen me have a seizure not only once (something that could be passed off as an accident or misfortune) but repeatedly; there was now no denying that seizures had to do with who I was. Knowing intellectually that the prejudice inside and outside was wrong helped me make up my mind while walking across the emergency room lobby that I was walking back in as a physician and would work as a physician just like on any other day. I tried to show the confidence and comfort on my face of knowing I belonged and to hide the fear and doubts in my heart.

Helen was the first to come up to me, and her concern was clear.

"Are you okay?"

Helen was not questioning my ability to return. She was worried about whether I had again bled into my head. Other nurses followed her lead and showed nothing but kindness. They treated me just like any one of the many people with medical problems they encounter every day. I have no knowledge of what discussions, if any, took place in my absence.

I sat down at the computer terminal and punched in my own patient number to look up my laboratory test results. The Tegretol level in my blood had been adequate.

After the first day, I did not hesitate as much at the door when I entered the emergency department, but it took several days of being the doctor and not the patient before I entered unpreoccupied.

CHAPTER TEN

Not Enough Time for Patients' Needs

W HILE I WAS on the wards, Dr. Barrows asked me to schedule another MRI, one of several since the surgery. Each time the MRI was repeated—since the first postoperative MRI, when everyone was certain but everyone disagreed—the radiologists said they did not know whether the vascular tumor remained. Each time, they suggested that the MRI be repeated in a few months, when they might know for sure.

In the radiology suite, a glass-topped wall separated where I lay in the large Magnetic Resonance Imager from where the radiologist sat on a high chair by a control panel. At the end of the test, a nurse came into the room containing the imager, pressed the button that conveyed patients flat on their backs out of the machine, took the hair net off my head, and said I could go.

"The doctor will call you with the results," she added.

I hesitated at the door to the room where the radiologist sat in front of a computer looking at the images of my brain as they flashed across the screen. The distance between us remained as impassable as if there had been a real wall. He did not invite me in to look or offer any preliminary report of what he saw.

"Your doctor will be calling you about what we see," he said, trying to move me along.

But he was already seeing. Emboldened by having endured, I walked in, stood beside him, and began to look at the screen. My face immediately became expressionless as I faced for the first time the hole that had been left in my brain after the surgery. Brain tissue is varying shades of gray on an MRI, and bones are white. There in between the tissue and bone on my MRI lay a small jet-black area empty of anything but fluid. The radiologist asked again that I talk to Dr. Barrows to learn about what the MRI showed.

By Sunday I was anxious about the Monday meeting with Dr. Barrows, about asking what was left of the cavernous hemangioma? What did the hole represent? What was my prognosis now? What were the statistics on risks to any children I might have? Thinking about the last question was one of the few things that still made me cry.

"The hemangioma is all gone," Dr. Barrows said before I could even sit down.

It was hard not to be silenced by disbelief. He had said only part was removed — some remained — with equal conviction so many times.

"How are you doing?" he asked, as I stared at him.

"Fine. Working hard," I said, giving the expected response. "The only thing I've noticed is that I have a hard time understanding words that I hear only with my left ear — like on the phone at work. Could that be at all related to the surgery?"

"No, I really doubt it," he replied.

"What's missing from that black hole?" I asked, pointing at the MRI, which was posted on a radiologic light box in Dr. Barrows's office. I wondered if the hole was the source of the problem.

"That's just where the hemangioma was. If you have any

more questions, you can always give me a call," he concluded kindly but cutting conversation short.

As I walked down an old, metal back staircase, his words kept replaying. I did not know what to believe anymore. I felt like the child in the story of the emperor's new clothes, who is told that only the wise can see the elegance of the clothes; the naive think he is naked.

After the appointment with Dr. Barrows I returned to work at Children's Hospital to the busiest admissions day of my internship year. Still, it was like coming up for a gasp of air after a long swim under water. I prayed my grandfather's prayer, which he translates from a language that he no longer remembers: "Thank you, God, for these blessings; please, God, do not take them away."

I talked to my father on the phone. He was perplexed. "I'm not sure I understand," he said. "The seizures are still not under control. You still have to take anticonvulsants." He stopped just short of completing the thought: I'm not sure why the new findings make any difference. Neither of the original goals — coming off anticonvulsants for a safer pregnancy or preventing seizures for safer work overseas — had been met. But my expectations had long since decreased, and at least the specter of future bleeds seemed to be diminished.

After phoning Tim and my parents with the apparent good news, I went downstairs to the emergency room.

In June I began to work on the cardiology service with three other interns. Our first morning, it was made clear to us that we should not make any decisions about patient care on weekdays. All medical decisions, including the most routine, were made by fellows, who had had four years of training after graduating from medical school, if not by attending physicians themselves. Setting the dose of some medications can be a complex art form, of others formulaic. Monday through Friday on the cardiology service, fellows determined the dosages, even of medications that were formulaic, and interns did the paperwork.

Instead of there being a system in which interns exercised increasing responsibility under gradually decreasing supervision, interns went from having little responsibility on weekdays to having little supervision at night, on weekends, and on holidays. When the interns were on call, there were often neither attendings nor fellows on the floor. Interns would make decisions not only about straightforward medication orders but also about life-threatening conditions. The difference between weekends and weekdays had the potential to endanger patients.

On the Memorial Day holiday, I was left alone to start my first day on call for the cardiology service. From the end of rounds at 10:00 A.M. until 11:00 P.M. that night, I saw the cardiology fellow out of the intensive care unit for only thirty-second intervals in the hall. Minutes after I arrived, a nurse came running to find the physician on call. Sammy was in respiratory distress. Finding that the oxygen saturation of his blood had dropped to 63 percent (normal is between 98 percent and 100 percent), I ordered oxygen, did a physical exam, got a chest X ray, and noted that his breath sounds were decreased on the right side. The fellow later came in and agreed with these steps. Then he rapidly returned to the intensive care unit, where he needed to care for several children who were walking a thin line between life and death, and left me once again with a ward of thirty children about whom I knew little.

That was typical of interns' experiences in cardiology throughout the year. Although the patients on the cardiology service were far sicker than most patients on the wards, supervision on weekends was available only when the patients in the intensive care unit were stable enough for the cardiology fellow to spare a few moments.

The fellows were committed both to teaching and patient care but had been forced to choose between caring for children who might die at any minute and supervising care for children who were desperately ill but not likely to die that night. The answer to any questions about those children whose lives were not immediately threatened was always "We'll be able to discuss that later."

The following year, supervision would be improved by the hiring of an additional cardiology fellow.

On rounds we were taught to listen carefully for heart murmurs that were quieter than a whisper. At the same time, we were taught by example to block out the silenced cries of parents. It was not by choice that the fellows spent little time listening to and talking with the parents. They simply had no time; they were caring for too many critically ill children, some of whom might die if left uncared for during a conversation.

The parents slept in foldout chairs at their children's bedsides. No one ever discussed, and I never fully understood until years later, when I returned to Children's Hospital as a parent, what it meant to try and cope with the sadness and fear of having a sick child while constantly being kept awake by four children in one shared room who woke each other up in a round robin as they cried in pain and fear for their mothers. The parents of children with severe congenital heart disease had to face incomparably more.

So many of the families of children on the cardiology service faced repeatedly life-threatening illness. Eddie had been living at home with aortic stenosis, a critical narrowing of a valve in his heart. He was being watched by his cardiologist until he was old enough to have the valve surgically repaired. The day he came to the hospital, he had been seen by his cardiologist. An echocardiogram showed that the difference in pressure across his aortic valve was more than 100 mm of mercury — a difference high enough to cause Eddie's heart to stop suddenly. His parents were instructed to take Eddie to the hospital right away, and they went straight to the hospital from their doctor's office without even stopping for clothes or formula. I can only imagine that his father's face showed the same pale terror, the same hauntingly desperate look for answers that it would have when his son's heart arrested. As doctors and nurses flooded in to try and revive Eddie, parents of the three other children who shared the room were shunted out. As they worried about their own children, these parents stood silently by, watching Eddie's mother pace the hallway and his father sit crumpled in a chair. Closed doors did not block out the shouts of the code and the sounds of the attempts to shock the toddler's heart back into action.

It was late when I finally met Betsy and her mother. Betsy's mother had received more than forty units of blood for uncontrollable bleeding after Betsy's birth. Eventually only a hysterectomy saved her life. She ended up with chronic hepatitis from one of the transfusions, the knowledge that she could have no future pregnancies, and a child with an uncertain survival due to complex heart disease.

"It took a year before I recovered," Betsy's mother began. "Not so much physically as emotionally. I spent a lot of time angry and upset about why I could not have any more children when there were so many people who could have them but didn't want them . . ."

As I sat on the end of the bed listening to her talk, I thought about the stages each of us goes through when forced to live with physical losses as dramatic as hers, and about how ill-prepared doctors are to deal with their patients' grief. Doctors receive little training in handling the process of grieving when a patient is dying and none at all when the patient is not terminally ill but is grieving over the changes and losses in her life. With far smaller losses than Betsy's mother's, I had gone through periods similar to hers — denial, anger, and bargaining — before reaching acceptance.

On the weekends, EKG's had to be performed, IV's placed, blood drawn — all by the intern, leaving even less time to care for the thirty patients who were on the ward with serious heart conditions. The support staff available on weekdays to place intravenous lines and draw blood were not at work.

We caught a glimpse of what might happen if future changes in the American health care system lead to fewer support staff on the wards. The understaffing of physicians, phlebotomists, and technicians and the need to care for the sickest children first meant that there was too little time to care for the children who were admitted for "elective procedures," including catheterization of their hearts.

The Miranda family was not seen by any physician — attending, fellow, or resident — for half a day after arriving in the hospital. Their one-year-old, Gabriela, already had such severe heart disease that her toenails had become bent purple clubs from lack of circulating oxygen. Her family, originally from Brazil, had taken her everywhere they could in search of a way to save her life. She had had catheterizations in Colombia and Panama, but the only treatment she had received was "plenty of drinking water." They had been waiting six months, as her heart disease became more severe, for a chance to come to Children's Hospital.

I worried about what it must be like for parents who have traveled great distances to come into the hospital with their child the afternoon before a serious and frightening procedure and not see a doctor until the middle of the night, when she wakes them and their child up. Still, before seeing new families who had been waiting for hours, I had to care for a child who was breathing three times as fast as normal, so hard that her chest wall was hitting her back and her nostrils were flaring. With the understaffing there was no choice.

Some of the cuts that are made to streamline expenses are far from cost-free to patients. There is no doubt they look better on paper than in person.

Not having enough time to provide the best care was a problem on other medical and surgical services as well.

Marcos had stopped using his right arm. At nine months, children cannot explain what is wrong, which joint hurts or whether the pain radiates, but they do not fake symptoms. When Marcos's X ray came back, it showed a bony lesion suspicious of cancer. Marcos's mother was a single parent with no one to support her in the emergency room. We had to tell her our concerns so that a bone marrow biopsy could be done.

When I began to explain the possible diagnosis to her, she just looked straight ahead. "There's a chance it might be cancer, but even if it is cancer, there are many treatments we can offer Marcos . . ." It took several minutes for my words to sink in before she suddenly burst out crying. We held each other and talked for the next half hour.

Then the cancer specialist came in and asked her permission to do a bone marrow biopsy. He did not know whether the mother had heard that cancer was a possible diagnosis. In asking her permission he was perfunctory. He stood up across the room by the door during the whole conversation and completed the discussion in two and a half minutes.

This doctor went into pediatrics probably because he cares about children and their families as much as I do. As an intern, he might well have taken as long as I did to explain a problem;

my method was typical of the residents I observed. But now, as a fellow, he had no time to share with parents, only enough time to perform procedures. Throughout the health care system, physicians are highly rewarded — both in prestige and payments — for performing procedures. The incentives for spending less and less time with patients are strong.

While on the cardiology service, I continued to see outpatients in my weekly clinic. In the beginning of the year, all appointments with interns were scheduled for an hour — more than four times as long as typical primary care appointments in much of the country — to allow enough time for the intern to learn. I kept as many hour-long appointments as I could throughout the year so I could talk at length with my patients and their parents.

Ali's mother, Janis, often booked the last appointment of the day. With no other patients waiting, we could spend even longer than scheduled talking in the small room with its plain examining table, small desk, and two hard plastic chairs that could have been taken out of an elementary school classroom. Ali had difficulty sleeping. At six, she still slept in bed with her mother and often urinated in the bed at night. She had been living in a neighborhood with nightly shootings. Even after moving to a safer neighborhood, she still did not know if she could trust the world around her.

Most of us do not reveal our hearts in five minutes. When our problem is complicated, it can rarely be solved in another five. Even if it could, that would leave only two minutes of an average twelve-minute appointment for a physical exam and such preventive care as vaccinations. Health care in the United States, frequently structured and financed around short visits, is designed to discourage discussions between patients and doctors. When I was thinking about the work I would do after residency, I worried about where I could practice pediatrics and continue to spend a lot of time with each patient, as I did in my clinic. The primary care pediatricians I knew were often constrained to spending only five to fifteen minutes with each patient — even when they felt it was important to spend more.

When I returned from clinic, Jonathan was waiting to be admitted. At birth, he had had a relatively simple problem: a blood vessel that is open in fetuses but that is supposed to shut at birth had not closed. The difficulty identifying the vascular anatomy of a newborn during surgery makes it hard to correct the problem. Instead of clipping the vessel, the surgeons had severed a main artery to one of Jon's lungs. The error was not detected for more than a year, by which time injuries to the affected lung were permanent.

Jonathan's mother told me that no one informed her of the surgical mistake for months after it was discovered; I was stunned. Later, students would tell me of their own experiences of physicians hiding errors from patients. In one typical story, a patient at another hospital needed to stay in the hospital for two months because a mistake the surgeons had made led to devastating infections. No one told the patient that the surgical error caused the complications. When I met Jonathan, I had not yet realized how common it was for silence to surround mistakes, even when the silence had serious consequences for the patient's health.

Nor did I know that in May a mistake in my care had been confirmed. When the pathologist changed his findings to report that blood vessels, not a hemangioma, had been removed during my surgery, neither the pathologist nor Dr. Barrows called.

Preparing to go to work on the next to last Friday of the cardiology rotation, I was so tired that I fell asleep standing up and dropped my Cheerios. The loud clatter of the bowl startled me and woke me up. The year had taught me patience, a patience that became as ingrained as the fatigue. So instead of swearing I just quietly picked up all the Cheerios.

Later that day, as I sat and listened to the discussion at the noon medical teaching conference, I noticed that my left hand, lying in front of me next to an uneaten sandwich on the table, was beginning to jerk. I grabbed my left hand with my right and unsuccessfully tried to hold it still; the jerking motion spread to my entire left lower arm. I used my right arm to swing my left arm under the table, where it would not alarm anyone.

Within a minute, the movements subsided. I retraced each stage in my mind, trying to test whether it had been a localized seizure. The fantasy that it was not, that I was not continuing to have seizures, was erased as I walked back to the ward at the end of the conference and the left side of my face began to twitch. It, too, subsided without generalizing, but with it went any remaining denial.

This time I was not sick, only tired. That night I went straight to sleep and slept most of the next day. It had been a year since my first seizure. At least these seizures were only focal ones.

CHAPTER ELEVEN

Patients' Families

LATER IN THE SUMMER, together with two other interns, I was given an orientation to work in the intensive care
unit and shown where the equipment for emergencies was located. As interns, we were ready for the pace of the medical
care in the ICU. Over and over interns are taught just to worry
about the ABC's, that to survive the patient needed to have a
patent *A*irway — if he did not have one, then make one — to
*B*reathe — if she was not breathing, then breathe for her — and
to have *C*irculation — if his blood was not circulating, then
move it with chest compressions. In the hospital, by the time the
ABC's were being addressed, a full-code team would arrive.

Furthermore, the nurses and respiratory therapists were
always at the bedside of patients in the ICU and were ready to
train new residents each month. If an intern was spending too
much time getting a history of a patient's high blood pressure
and considering whether it was from withdrawal of a medicine,
they would quickly remind him, "A mean arterial blood pressure of eighty is considered critically high," and ask, "How
about some hydralazine?" letting you know the urgency of the
decision and suggesting what to give the patient.

But we were not prepared for the personal side of the repeated, rapidly evolving tragedies.

My first day on call in the ICU I spent time with each family there. Katie lay below photographs of what she had been like before she got sick and beside the teddy bear that she could no longer even reach for. Her condition had been critical when she arrived at the hospital. Her kidneys had shut down, and she had stopped urinating altogether.

After three days in the hospital, she had finally begun to urinate again. She had opened her eyes, then gradually responded to voices, fixing her eyes on people and following them. Her mother sat alone in the parent area, afraid of seeing the daughter who looked so good to us and so bad to her. I went to bring the news that Katie could try to drink again. Her mother sat back hesitantly.

"You can hold her and feed her."

No response.

"I'm sure it'll be special for her that it's you," I suggested, thinking that many parents, after some initial hesitancy, feel better when they can hold and nourish their own child.

No movement.

"Would you like to come be with her?"

"When?"

"Now."

Later that night, Katie's father arrived with his second wife. It was his first time seeing Katie in the hospital. He spoke with anger heightened by fear and remorse, without looking at Katie's mother: "We usually have Katie on the weekends. We were told last Saturday she was away for the weekend. We didn't get here sooner because we had no idea . . ."

"We did go away," her mother began to explain listlessly. "When we got home, she started to feel sick . . . diarrhea . . . like a stomach bug. . . ."

The stress of sick children did not widen only preexisting fault lines within families. The stress also fractured well-functioning relationships.

But at times, the strains caused by a child's critical illness renewed old alliances. Annie started losing her developmental milestones at seven months. Now, as a two-year-old, all she had left were uncontrolled, eerie dancelike movements around a collar that held in place the tube that went through her neck into her windpipe. Her eyes were open with a vacant stare, unable to follow anyone. Her mouth was still. The last smile was long gone.

The intensive care unit was a large room with only curtains separating patients' beds. An alarm went off as Annie's heart rate dropped. The nurse turned the alarm off as the medical team stood at a nearby patient's bed. As we continued to walk around the beds on afternoon rounds, our eyes kept going back to Annie. When we arrived at her bedside, Annie's nurse immediately asked, "What's her status?"

"She doesn't have one yet."

"You should really get a DNR before something happens," she advised.

Annie had just been bathed, and smelled only of the ointment used to prevent diaper rash and the disinfectant used to keep her intravenous and arterial lines from becoming infected. She was being given "comfort measures": tube-fed, talked to, and handheld. There was nothing more anyone could do. Annie's brain had gradually deteriorated over the previous two years. Tests repeated that day had confirmed that her heart had become so diseased from the same degenerative process that her death was imminent. The entire team agreed that if her heart stopped, resuscitation efforts would only mean a painful prolongation of her death.

In the ICU, the resident on call carries out the patient

care decisions that have been made by the team on afternoon rounds. I was on call but only an attending can write an order not to resuscitate a patient. So I went to ask John Weld, the attending in charge of the ICU for the day, to discuss the possibility of a DNR status with Annie's parents.

Just that morning, Dr. Weld had given a conference on caring for patients at the end of life. The messages in his lecture had been clearly written on the blackboard. "When death is imminent, it is often appropriate not to take extraordinary measures to prolong the course of an incurable terminal illness"; "Decide with a patient's family what to do before the patient's heart stops beating or the patient stops breathing"; "Written DNR orders are important."

Recalling the lecture and knowing his detailed familiarity with each patient's condition, I anticipated that Dr. Weld would understand immediately why it was important to speak with Annie's family. But he found a thousand excuses.

"I want to wait until next week when genetics gives us more information for the family," he began, in the first of many attempts to excuse himself, professionally placing the responsibility on others.

But I knew that while the information we had gathered was valuable to inform future pregnancies, the test results would not alter Annie's prognosis. Her heart had shown a rapid irreversible deterioration on repeated echocardiograms. I was worried about what would happen if her heart stopped before a meeting was scheduled the following week, so I pressed Dr. Weld.

Still resisting, he continued, "You don't need a written DNR in the ICU. Everyone is a potential DNR." But that was painfully untrue in practice. A DNR decision needs to be made before the moment of death.

As a medical student, I had witnessed just what happens

when everyone agrees on a DNR status but one is not written. An elderly man had had two different primary cancers. He was dying of widely metastatic disease and was already in his late eighties, but no DNR order had been written. Instead, the attending asked that when the man had an arrest he be called and he would advise that resuscitation was not medically indicated. The man's heart stopped, and we called the attending, but the attending was stuck in traffic in a tunnel and was unable to answer his page. Consequently, chest compressions were begun, and the patient was shocked electrically many times in an effort to get his heart beating again. He was aggressively resuscitated for an hour before he was revived, entirely comatose, permanently unresponsive, having gone through a long series of painful procedures that would bring him no more meaningful life.

"We can't write a DNR order without the mother here," Dr. Weld continued.

"But her father has offered to call her mother," I said, explaining that she could be at Children's Hospital in three hours.

"I don't want to call her when there's nothing imminent. This decision can wait. And I don't want to approach her parents for the first time on a Friday afternoon."

But, I thought, they'll be here all weekend. Every day was the same in their vigil of grief. It was Friday afternoon only for him.

The decision practically and legally rested with the attending on duty. I walked to Annie's bedside. When I arrived, the nurse said, "Annie's father's just told me he's been waiting for four hours for an attending to discuss a DNR status with him in the parents' room." It surprised me that Annie's father had thought he had a noon appointment, since none of the medical staff knew about it, but it was no surprise that he had thought about a DNR status or that he was ready to talk about his decision. Most parents who have been through long illnesses with terminally ill children have thought at length about it, although some are not as ready to make the decision. I paged John Weld, and Jim Samuels answered. "I'm on call for Dr. Weld," he said. Dr. Weld had left for the weekend five minutes after my last conversation with him. Dr. Samuels spoke quietly with Annie's father and his fiancée alone in the parents' room. Then together they called Annie's mother. Jim Samuels wrote the DNR order.

Annie's parents were separated, but they had spoken to each other about Annie's status to make sure they were in agreement. The afternoon of the decision, her father drove north three hours to pick up Annie's mother and bring her back to the ICU. In fewer than three days Annie began to die. Because of the DNR order, when her heart stopped on its own, her parents were able to rock her in their arms in a wooden chair at her bedside and say good-bye.

Everyone had agreed that Annie's prognosis was abysmal. That was part of what made the decision that she should be DNR as straightforward as any such decision can be. If patients' prognoses were always as clear as Annie's, medical practice would be entirely different. The often quoted figures of how much money and effort is spent on caring for people in the last weeks of life don't take into account how poor we are at projecting when the last weeks of life have begun. Disagreements about prognoses are magnified by the stakes.

Danielle's father had been through countless admissions of his daughter. Now Danielle lay wasted in her ICU bed, fourteen years old and fifty-four pounds. Her father stayed at her side. Danielle's kidneys had been destroyed by disease before she even entered school. The years that followed included dialysis, transplant, rejection, waiting for another transplant, and again kidney failure. She was running out of options.

Then Danielle had a cardiac arrest. She was unable to talk

or respond to people afterward. As it became gradually clear that the chances were vanishing that medical care could do anything to make it possible for her to survive — let alone speak, move, or live outside the hospital again — discussions began about how much more should be tried to prolong her life and when she should be allowed to die. Everyone participated — her family, more than a dozen past and present health caregivers — everyone except Danielle, who could no longer even acknowledge a visitor's presence. Some of the doctors and nurses had known Danielle since she looked like the happy girl in the picture that hung over her bed. Those of us who had only seen her desperately ill held less hope that she would recover. Danielle's father's whole life was wrapped up in her. His son, Sam, had already died.

Danielle herself, when she was still able to talk, had been ready to let go. On the hospital ward, before she had grown so sick that she was transferred to the ICU, she had told her father she was going to die. When her father tried to disagree, Danielle said, "Don't worry, Dad. I know I'm dying. It's okay. I want to see Sam."

A nurse came into the dark of the on-call room at 4:00 A.M. "Danielle is tachycardic." Her heart was beating several times its normal pace.

"I'll be right there." I ran to her bed as I tried to replace the dreams in my mind with the reality of medicine. The ICU team spent the next four hours stabilizing Danielle.

The culture of medicine has many myths based on the mistaken reasoning that just because physicians respond to the suffering they see, they are not affected by it. While some emergency professionals have designed group gatherings to support each other in dealing with the effects of their work on themselves, doctors do next to nothing. Discussing difficult experiences is often taken as a sign of weakness. It is acceptable to discuss physical fatigue from on-call schedules but not the emotional weariness that comes from dealing with death. But doctors are no less vulnerable to the flashbacks that serve as reminders of horrors survived. How physicians try to live with what we have lived through may have a marked effect on both our own lives and how we treat patients.

Tim and I both felt the effects of our experiences, as did our colleagues. Tim can joke and laugh through any situation, and his lightheartedness made him stand out during his internship and residency. But the horrors he saw were not hidden from him in his dreams. During Tim's internship, I woke up once in the middle of the night to find him going through the motions of intubating me in his sleep. As I shook him, trying to wake him, he called out, "We need help! We need help! The patient in Room Eight is not breathing. Get me an intubation tray!" I shook him and finally roused him from the depths of his day.

In the intensive care unit, my dreams were vivid: Endo was two years old, but as small as a premature baby. Having reached few developmental milestones, he had now completely regressed neurologically. He could no longer recognize anyone. He could no longer see. He could no longer smile. His family had finally decided to let him die. His father, standing by his side, was a physician. He had agreed that after Endo died, his body would be used to teach resuscitation before he was put to rest. He had agreed, but I had not. As we resuscitated Endo's dead body, knowing there was no hope, everything went wrong. We were in another hospital's emergency ward, and all the bags used for resuscitation were different from our own and antiquated. We could not get air into Endo's body. It was not supposed to matter because he had died. But it did matter. The exercise was repeated again and again, each time with a new resident. As I got increasingly distraught, the father repeated too blandly what I had heard many other physicians say: "Well, there are some really horrible things we have to do to people as doctors." After the third resuscitation exercise, I offered Endo's mother, as we are taught to do after a death, the chance for a last moment alone. We handed poor Endo's body to her to hold. Endo was limp and lifeless. Then, all of a sudden, his eyes began to move. He began to become alert and said, "Mama, Mama, Mama." Then I woke up to hear Ben shouting, "Mommy, Mommy, Mommy," his call having breathed the life into the child in my dream.

The dream came from one child's life and another child's death. It came from the stories others had told me during medical school of being taught to intubate on a dead patient and from an attending's advice that we learn the technique of placing emergency intravenous lines on patients who had died. It came from having watched a parent tell the story of her daughter's death blandly, as she stood watching the resuscitation in shock. The dream came from disbelief in the pretense that physicians present that they are not affected by death. It came from the horrors that physicians inflict in trying to save their patients and from the horrors their patients go through when they are ready to die in peace. It came from how little we know about when anybody is ready to die.

Whoever describes death as a peaceful falling asleep is not describing any of the deaths I witnessed in children. Their parents, their brothers and sisters, their caretakers were rarely ready to give them up. Even when a child had a DNR status, the pulse of the pain was palpable long after the patient's was not. When the death was sudden, the wailing and the railing at the world — at its unfairness, at the randomness of events — overshadowed every other sound. One preschool boy, struck by a car as he crossed the street just steps ahead of his parents, lay with tubes coming out of every orifice and limb, needle marks everywhere from our desperate attempts to reverse the irreversible. Resuscitations of children often went long, long past the point when there was any more hope. I continued to pray because I had to pray.

Families play crucial roles in patients' lives from admission to recovery or death. Philip's family got him to the hospital in time. The youngest of five boys, Philip had learned not to speak about pain. His silence about his pain hid the severity of his condition. Philip had been put in a regular emergency department room, not one of the three reserved for those patients known to need the most rapid care. The triage nurse did not even write "Urgent" by his name. He had fallen from the football tackles the day before. Still in elementary school, he had been practicing on the high school equipment. The impression at triage must have been that since he had been well enough to go home after his injury, spend the night there, and come back by car, not ambulance, this must be a routine post-fall check. When I entered the room, his heart was racing. Within moments, so was mine.

Philip began to talk in a quiet voice as his older brothers surrounded him. During the night, each time he had tried to walk to the bathroom, he had begun to faint. His belly had become increasingly painful. As he continued to talk, I began to examine his abdomen. As I placed my hands gently on his belly, he squeezed his eyes closed against the pain and grew silent. I pressed down slowly and gently, then released my hands all at once. He cried out for the first time. He had marked rebound tenderness, a sign that the lining of his belly was inflamed from bleeding. I explained that I would be bringing in other physicians and quickly went to alert the senior physicians in the emergency room to Philip's condition and to ask the nurses to set up for a large-bore intravenous line. Treatment had to begin immediately.

In the care of dependent children and adults, it is often the parent, sibling, spouse, or adult child who makes the critical decision when to seek help. Some children were brought in for small cuts, but Philip had spent the night at home with a major, though veiled, abdominal injury. Two of Philip's four brothers came into his room. His brothers had wanted to bring Philip to the emergency room during the night. They were angry because their father had said, "No, no. Wait until morning and see." But collectively the family had decided to bring Philip to the hospital — in time to save his life.

Philip did not flinch as several intravenous lines were placed. He began to express his pain and fear on the way to the intensive care unit.

At the end of work once a week, I went regularly to physical therapy to correct muscular damage wrought by the length of the neurosurgery. When my appetite began to return after surgery, it became clear that I could not open my mouth more than an inch. It was summertime; I could not eat corn on the cob. Nor could I eat apples, bananas, or bread crusts unless they were made into mush. I spoke to Dr. Barrows on the phone. He said that it was a muscular injury and that it would go away on its own.

Eight months later, when the oral surgeon was evaluating my jaw, he lamented that neurosurgeons so often ignore the problem of postoperative scarring of the muscles. Caught early, the repair is easy; caught late, the repair is difficult and far less promising. When I called Dr. Barrows, an easy intervention would have been available; I was far from the first patient whose voice had gone unheard.

By spring, the muscles had scarred down. To correct the

damage would require either further surgery, with no guarantee of success, or extensive physical therapy. I had had enough surgery.

One Friday afternoon, I was walking with hunched shoulders, every muscle aching, to the physical therapist's office. I was so exhausted that as soon as I touched the table I fell asleep. As Sarah, the physical therapist, moved my jaw open and closed through painful maneuvers, I slept. She woke me up at the end and sent me home. I fell asleep again on the subway despite trying my hardest to keep my eyes open in order not to miss my stop.

That week, Danielle's father had walked in as we were intubating her. The mother of a second patient had chanted Haitian prayers at the bedside of her daughter, hoping to revive her more completely than the medical team had been able to after a near-fatal accident. A third child had almost drowned in a ditch after a car accident on the way home from her grandmother's birthday. A fourth child's father was released from jail to come visit his unconscious son. The hospital guards had to take him away when he shouted at and threatened the staff after looking on helplessly, not knowing whether to believe the system was providing the best care it could. And that was just the beginning.

On the subway, I dreamt that Samantha, an infant on the surgical service who was dying from a diaphragmatic hernia that had caused irreparable damage to her lungs, had survived. As I reached home after being at work for thirty-six hours, my thoughts slowing through the haze of sleep deprivation, I could not pretend to leave work behind. I was worrying about Danielle and what condition she and her father were in as Ben climbed up on me, protesting any attempts at sleep since it had been a day and a half since he had seen me.

CHAPTER TWELVE

Embracing Life

SINCE ENTERING MEDICAL SCHOOL, I had hoped to combine patient care with work on health policy. During internship I was awarded a MacArthur Foundation Fellowship to conduct health policy research at Harvard. The fellowship would allow me to conduct research, and complete a Ph.D. in public policy, but I would not be able to see patients at the same time. As the year came to a close, I was ambivalent, excited about beginning the fellowship yet deeply saddened by the prospect of saying good-bye to patients.

When residents leave Children's, their clinic patients are transferred to the care of other physicians. I sat with other residents around a conference table reading medical charts and writing transfer notes. Marc's chart gave me sorrowful pause.

Marc's deep brown eyes were handsome despite their sadness when we met the day he was born. He was born shaking, and he shook for days, withdrawing from the drugs he had become addicted to in the womb. Unlike healthy babies, the second anyone touched him, he jumped. He would go from a deep sleep to a screaming cry at a moment's notice. We had called in the Department of Social Services (DSS) from the neonatal intensive care unit. DSS had been involved with his mother before. She had abused Marc's older siblings.

"We'll have a social worker follow the family," the representative from DSS explained.

"For how long?"

"For at least the first couple weeks."

"How often will someone see them?" I asked, worried about the short duration of the visits.

"Probably once a week, depending on the social worker's schedule."

"Will there be any drug treatment program for the mom?"

"Only if she needs it. She says she doesn't use drugs regularly. She says she tried them once, the night before Marc was born, and that's why he tested positive."

"But then he wouldn't have been born addicted."

Marc would be particularly challenging to care for as he went through withdrawal from addiction in the womb. He might well have incurred permanent disabilities from the drug exposure, yet he was to be sent home to a mother who had abused her other children, who had been using cocaine during her pregnancy, and who had not been through a treatment program. She would have only a couple of perfunctory visits by social services. If Marc and his mother could be helped together, it was not by two short visits. It was by a drug treatment program and extensive follow-up.

Social services has swung like a pendulum from believing that children should rapidly be removed from abusive families to believing that endless efforts should be made to keep any family together. Both strategies have drawbacks for the same reason that universal medical recommendations do: they do not adequately consider differences among those being served. Although many families fall into a gray zone, there are some who would clearly be able to care for their children if given adequate support services, and there are others in which abuse is so severe that it is hard to imagine it could be stopped without separation. Furthermore, DSS is desperately understaffed; done right, "family preservation" is labor-intensive.

Each of my clinic patients' lives was as profoundly affected by health and social policy as by their medical care. Providing care in the hospital, I could help Marc in the neonatal intensive care unit, but not before he became addicted in the womb. During clinic visits, Ali's mother and I bore witness to the impact of violence in her neighborhood, but I could not dent the circumstances she faced. On Team C, I could care for Katrina but do nothing to prevent her from developing AIDS. It was to work on health and social policy that I was accepting the MacArthur Foundation Fellowship. For the first two years at Harvard, my focus would be research aimed at limiting the spread of AIDS and tuberculosis. After two years, I would expand the range of my work to include other areas of children's health and the problem of access to health and social services. Dr. Feder and Dr. Weissman, who ran the training program, were strongly supportive of my plans.

When physicians at Children's asked what I would be doing next, I explained that I would begin work on AIDS and tuberculosis. While I frequently received support, the answer was at times met with contempt. One of the attendings, Phil Earls, a laboratory researcher, searched his memory for someone who had done anything that seemed to him remotely similar. He contended, "I have a friend who did that. He worked for USAID trying to solve the garbage problem in Cairo, and it was a complete bust." He felt strengthened in his certainty of its worthlessness.

The disdain some senior physicians show for anyone who works in the area of health policy or public health is problematic because it discourages undecided physicians-in-training from entering the fields at a time when the need is great. Preventable illnesses and injuries are the leading causes of death of children and young adults; 40 million Americans are without health insurance and often without primary care. Still, some doctors find it incomprehensible that any competent professional would want to work on these problems. Tony Nelson, a cardiologist who taught pathology, would warn us, "You need to learn it if you're going to be a *real* doctor. Some people never learn it; they have to go run a community health center."

My internship ended under the ceaselessly bright fluorescent emergency room lights in the middle of the last night of September. Jessy, a large, muscular young African-American man, was simultaneously fighting sickness and stereotype. The nurse caring for him had told me that he had been uncooperative bordering on belligerent. She had seen him just seconds before I did and said he refused to tell her anything about how he was feeling, who his doctor was, what medications he was taking, or what his medical history was. She knew he had been brought in by ambulance after an apparent seizure.

When I saw him, he lay on the emergency room bed, clearly post-ictal, in that state of confusion that follows a generalized seizure. He tried to answer questions but was not yet able to do so. As soon as the seizure and his confusion passed, he readily answered.

When the ambulance had come to get me after my first seizure, I had been treated as a drug addict. Although the discrimination differed, it cut across race and class. Ambulance drivers and nurses commonly see patients who have had seizures; more than two million Americans have epilepsy. The nurse should have recognized that Jessy was post-ictal, confused, and unable to respond.

That Sunday night in September, walking out of the hospital through the near-empty midnight halls, I stopped to hug fellow residents who were working. The 1950s juke box was still playing in the lobby, but the paging operator on duty had locked herself in the communications office for security. I knocked softly, then louder, finally needing to pound for her to open the door and accept my beeper.

Arriving home, I woke Tim up and danced. The next morning, I began work on a project with the World Health Organization. The World Health Organization's Global Programme on AIDS had invited me to work with it examining how a vaccine or cure for AIDS, if found, could be made available worldwide. In the case of Hepatitis B, an infection that kills millions worldwide, there had been almost a decade of delay between the availability of an effective vaccine in industrialized countries and the availability in developing countries where many more people suffered from the disease.

The night before I left for the World Health Organization's Geneva offices, my mother called.

Her first words were "Jody, do you think you're going to die young?" Even for my mother, who is never slow to get to the point, this was an abrupt beginning.

"No, I don't think I'm going to die any sooner because of what's happened." Then, after pausing, retreating slightly to ensure I was on the solid ground of truth on which our relationship rested: "We both know there are increased risks from having seizures and working in areas without health care, but I don't think they're that great."

After my first seizure and surgery, the distance between life and death had never again seemed wide. Over the course of the year my commitment to embracing each day had grown more quietly imbedded in each action and less an all-consuming mental monologue.

"You remember that in high school four friends my age died, and I dealt with it by trying to live my life as if each day were my last? I felt so strongly about it. Then, over the years, with most people living and counseling me to live in the future — medical school almost requiring it — I ended up living half in the present and half in the future. Well, now I have daily reminders of my vulnerability. I don't make any assumptions anymore about how long I'll live. I want to appreciate every day as if it were my last, to love the people I'm with, to show them my love, and to do as much as I can right now to contribute to the world." I did not continue because I knew that, although it had been painful to learn to live that way, it was almost trite to say.

Her call was just one more reminder that my life would never be exactly as it had been before, that I would not be able to say "I made it" or "I dealt with it" in the past tense. Only over time did I realize, then over even longer begin to accept, that my life had changed for the duration.

Enough time had passed since the surgery that the scar on the side of my head had turned white. A patch of skin, shaved for the surgery, was now covered with hair that curled around my ear.

Tim and I went to the fall semiformal for Children's Hospital residents. It was held in the top-floor restaurant of the Museum of Science, a plain cafeteria with a spectacular view overlooking the Charles River and the night lights of Boston.

Susan, who had worked in the outpatient clinic with me, came up to let me know about my patients and their parents. Hearing their news meant a lot to me. Like other patients and physicians who form strong attachments while working together, we greatly missed each other. Susan explained that Janis had called to ask if her daughter could still be my patient instead of transferring to a new doctor when I left Children's Hospital. Kahlila had decided to transfer to a different clinic. She had been taking time off from work for nearly a year to bring her son to his pediatric appointments with me. She would keep doing that if she could see me, she told them, but if she had to change pediatricians she would go to a clinic that had evening hours.

Tom had been an intern with me. He came up and interrupted Susan: "I couldn't believe you came back when you did, Jody." I was not sure which of the several "coming backs" he was referring to, so I just nodded as he went on to explain, fumbling for words, that he was not really sure how or why I did come back at all. I did not know what to say.

Then Jack came up.

"I'm in the NICU now. It's exciting doing deliveries, but the call's lousy. How are you?"

"I'm doing great."

"No, how are you really?" Then, when I looked confused, he added, "How is your health? Are you okay?" It was not that he asked about my health but that he could not believe I was doing well and felt bound at first to ask in code that made it clear he considered me and my life different from his own.

Other friends came up and repeated the same questions.

One can feel different or disabled in at least two ways: with respect to one's own life or condition in the past and with respect to the lives or conditions of others. It had taken me more than a year to come to the point where I did not believe my life would be seriously limited by my health. But after my life had begun to seem normal to me, it became clear that it did not seem normal to others. What I took as an illness no different from the variety of illnesses that any adult may suffer if she lives into middle and old age, some labeled as different, uniquely disabling, or stigmatizing.

I tried to visit a gym and the rules prohibited me from working out without the manager's permission because I had had seizures. I would have understood this had the management excluded all medical conditions that could lead to a loss of consciousness, but seizures were singled out.

When I answered a call for volunteers to donate bone marrow, I was told no one who had had seizures could be a donor. I thought with sadness of Gracey, a gentle, energetic five-year-old who was living in Children's Hospital in an isolation chamber with aplastic anemia, and of Sarah on the oncology ward, who had leukemia. Both were at risk of dying if a matched bone marrow donor could not be found soon. Not only were seizures in no way contagious, but these children's parents would surely have chosen epilepsy over death for their children in a flash if it had been contagious.

After the Children's Hospital dance, we gave Jerry and his brother a ride home. Jerry's brother mentioned that he was studying disabilities and had learned that children thought it would be worse to have a hidden disability than a visible one because they would have to keep explaining the disability.

The ranking of a wide range of aggregated disabilities does not make sense, but the idea that there is an important difference between visible and invisible disabilities does. I recalled flying alone to see my grandfather in Pittsburgh earlier that fall. After I sat down, I took out the metal orthopedic device that wrapped around my head and automatically opened and closed my jaw in order to redress the postsurgical scars. More disconcerting than the direct stares of the passengers was the flight attendant's response: she looked at everyone until she got to my row and then studiously averted her gaze as if looking at me was dangerous. With each pass, she simply found something important on her shoes to examine. She was embarrassed to look me in the eye, afraid that the interaction would be something other than human to human.

Epilepsy is often invisible. A stranger cannot see epilepsy

except during a seizure. Its unseen nature makes it harder to discriminate against people whose seizures are concealed, but that very concealment makes it easier to discriminate against those whose epilepsy is known.

The children were right that publicly disclosing and describing a disability that is subject to discrimination is difficult, and many adults have chosen not to. As a result, there are few voices to protest stereotypes about people who have seizures. Intertwined with invisibility is the inability to protest prejudice effectively.

Like polio, seizures can affect people for the first time in adulthood; both diseases have affected individuals who were well known before the onset of their health problem. In the case of polio, this has meant that there are public figures in a wide range of occupations who have been affected with visible post-polio disabilities. President Franklin Roosevelt had already been a New York state senator, secretary of the navy, and nominated vice president before having polio. FDR could hide neither his braces nor his difficulty walking.

But epilepsy can be hidden from anyone who is not present during a seizure. The public does not know which of our current intellectual, cultural, or political leaders has had seizures. Without that silence about who has had seizures, could discrimination have continued codified for so long in the United States? As recently as the 1960s, five states still had laws restricting marriage by persons with epilepsy; fourteen states authorized involuntary sterilization. North Carolina required sterilization before marriage.

In the context of this silence surrounding seizures, in November the *New England Journal of Medicine* published a review article in which the authors attributed significant psychosocial problems to those with epilepsy without citing a single reference on this point. It is impossible to imagine the *New*

England Journal of Medicine publishing a review article that said women have problems "building self-esteem" or that African-Americans have difficulty "establishing interpersonal relationships" without citing any research. But that is precisely what they did in describing people with seizures.

I responded in a letter to the editor:

> As a physician who has both treated patients with seizures and lived with seizures, I was disturbed by [the authors'] handling of the section on psychosocial issues. The authors' reference of physicians to the Epilepsy Foundation as an excellent resource for them and their patients is valuable. Unfortunately, this section also contains unintentionally misleading information, which has the potential to stoke the fire of prejudice as well as the belief from the Dark Ages that seizures are a form of mental illness.
>
> The authors state that "psychosocial dysfunction" is "often long-lasting" and occurs regardless of seizure control, yet give no data to support this. They go on to state "persons with epilepsy frequently have difficulty in establishing interpersonal relationships, building self-esteem, and obtaining or maintaining employment." Again in their otherwise well-referenced article, they take these statements for granted without calling on any well-conducted studies. Even if these statements were true, providing physicians with a meaningful approach to the problems would include a further analysis of whether the cause was the disease or social reaction. The remedy in one case is focused on the patient; the answer in the latter case includes attacking society's prejudices.
>
> I believe the authors' intention was to highlight the need for support services. Their goal of treating the whole patient with seizures and not "just the disease" was excellent. This is the approach we should take to patients with any type of disease. Having cared for families when their children were first diagnosed with seizures, I was aware of the importance of

providing support services both directly and by referral. Yet, I was also aware how important it was for the family to know that their child could lead a normal life, continue to form loving relationships and work productively in society, that their child could still be an athlete, a doctor, a lawyer, a writer, or a statesperson, as Dostoevski, Flaubert, Julius Caesar, and Emperor Charles V, to name a few, had before them.[1]

We should follow the advice that was given parents in an exceptional book on seizures: "You must understand the mythology and how different it is from reality. Only with this understanding can you avoid handicapping your child [or patient], prevent his being handicapped by others, and allow him to reach his full potential."[2]

Jody Heymann, M.D., M.P.P.
Harvard University

[1] Fisher RS. Seizure Disorders. In *Principles of Ambulatory Medicine,* ed. by Barker LR, Burton JR, and Zieve PD. Williams and Wilkins, 1986.

[2] Freeman JM, Vining EPG, Pillas DJ. Seizures and epilepsy in childhood: a guide for parents. Baltimore: Johns Hopkins Press, 1990. Parenthetical "or patient" added by author.

The *New England Journal of Medicine* published the letter with only four words removed. They would not print that I had lived with seizures, only that I had treated others.

During the fall of my first year as a MacArthur Foundation Fellow, I traveled alone to the World Health Organization in Geneva and to a meeting sponsored by the Rockefeller Foundation in Bellagio, Italy, to work on international AIDS prevention while Tim worked as a primary care physician. Tim and I wanted to celebrate what we had come through together during the past year and a half. We waited until January, until my parents could care for Ben and it was river-running season in Chile.

Tim and I had wanted to journey down the Bío-Bío in rural Chile, a river named after the song of a flycatcher. The Bío-Bío had been navigated for the first time only a dozen years earlier. River rapids are rated on a one-to-six scale, with one being flat water and six unnavigable. The Bío-Bío was filled with class five rapids. The area we would traverse included fifteen-foot holes.

Before my surgery, we had rafted the Paquare through the Costa Rican primordial forest. This time would be different. A part of my mind was now occupied with medications, with placing Tegretol in multiple waterproof containers scattered in different rafts so that if one raft flipped, there would still be enough dry medication to last the trip. There were no pharmacies along the way.

Four boats made the trip down the Bío-Bío together. Three boats were rowed by boatmen; each of these carried three passengers, who would hold on to ropes and gunnels as the boats were buffeted and battered by waterfalls and waterholes. Tim and I were in the fourth boat, which was propelled by passengers who paddled. The boatman would be our eyes; we would be his arms. All of us had picked the paddleboat because we wanted to work to get where we were going and to be able to feel the water as we went.

From one day to the next, the number and size of the rapids would grow until in one day we would paddle as many large rapids as boaters crossed in more than a week on the Colorado River. We would pull the rafts ashore and climb along the cliffs and rock-strewn banks of the river to scout the most dangerous rapids before trying to row them. All went easily until Lava South. Lava South was named after Lava Falls in the Grand Canyon, and both Lavas were among the hardest white water anywhere to navigate. As we entered, our raft flipped onto its side. As another paddler, Kyle, went overboard, my head went under water. As the raft righted, I pulled myself into it with my feet. Kyle made it to shore, breathless and shaken. After his fall, Kyle crouched closer to the center of the raft. We continued downriver beside hundred-foot waterfalls where tributaries entered.

We spent the days running rapids amid spectacular views of snowcapped peaks and lush green wilderness. Morning, noon, and night, we picnicked on the riverbanks and went swimming in calm eddies. We reached the rapid called One-Eyed Jack, around which the experts who first navigated the river had had to portage. Lower water made it navigable now as long as every part of the rapid was hit just right. But we went too close to an overhanging rock, where more than ten thousand cubic feet of water crashed each second. In the seconds we saw our raft flip over us, we prepared ourselves to swim the rapid feet first to protect our heads from the rocks. As soon as we were through the screaming water, we scrambled for eddies to avoid being swept into the rapids that lay immediately below and began the process of securing our raft out of the river. We fished for our gear as the wet bags floated downriver.

Between rapids, we spent a lazy layover day trying to keep our burned and blistering rowing hands out of the blazing sun. We gathered in the shade of a large tree, where the shadows of the leaves danced over our legs and where we were less disturbed by hundreds of sand-digging bees who sought the bright sunlight.

The next day, we set out to climb Mount Callaqui, a ten-thousand-foot active volcano. When we set out, I was not worried about the challenge. I had been climbing mountains for decades — as a child, three- and four-thousand-foot peaks in Vermont's Green Mountains, as an adult, rock- and glacier-covered seventeen-thousand-foot Mount Kenya. Each climb put me at peace with life. The solitude — even with friends — of climbing, of being surrounded by more clouds than people, brought solace as well as fatigue. The seizures had meant an end to the long peaceful swims I had once taken alone, hypnotized by the rhythm of breathing and watching sunlight dancing in the water. Mountains still seemed accessible.

On the first day, we hiked to a campsite at the base of the mountain, from which little of the mountain was visible. At four-thirty the following day in the predawn dark, we broke base camp so that we could make it to Callaqui's snowcapped top and back down again before the afternoon sun made avalanches and rock fall a real risk. Brad led us out at a rapid pace, pushing everyone's limits, wary of the afternoon risks. By breakfast at sunrise, I had fallen to last in line. I could barely breathe.

"Tim, I think I'm going to stop here," I gasped.

"What's wrong?"

"I can't breathe. . . . I'm wheezing. . . . so much," I choked out in short sentences while reaching for the Ventolin inhaler we carried in our pack. The cold air, altitude, and exertion had sent my bronchi into deep spasm. It was the first mountain I had climbed since developing asthma after pneumococcal pneumonia.

"I'll go back with you if you want," Tim offered.

"No, I'm fine. It won't be any problem going down slowly."

The Ventolin inhaler began to work. My breathing was still racing and shallow, my chest still tight with pain, but the desperate search for air was passing.

Kyle, who was hiking with us, turned around. "I want to go more slowly anyway. We could give it a try together."

"So do I," added Lisa.

So we formed a trio and one step at a time began to

climb. There were thousands of feet of scree, loose rock on which two steps forward were followed by one slide back, and a glacier to climb after the scree. Unless we dug our heels into the scree and snow, we risked sliding down far below where we had begun.

A half dozen times it looked as if we were almost there. But when we reached what looked like the top, we found only a local crest; much more of the mountain lay beyond. Finally we came to the smoking peak of the volcano.

Tim and John had reached the top first, hiking at a steady fast pace. Our trio arrived in the middle of the group, a three-legged turtle outpacing many hares.

From the top we could see the Andes and into Argentina. We could also see the other volcanoes in the ringlet of fire, including one which was named how I felt: Llaima, the reawakened one.

CHAPTER THIRTEEN

Snapshots: One and Two Years Later

LATE 1990 AND EARLY 1991

ROSSIE AND STEVE had been friends for years. At a lunch for just the three of us that Rossie set up, Steve asked many questions about seizures and about how they affected my life. He was still working through the issue of how adult onset seizures had affected his own.

Consciously from the start, before I had had any seizures in Children's Hospital, I took my anticonvulsant medications in public. It was a small statement, but I did not want to hide who I was. I talked openly about my seizures with friends. Still, it was hard to discuss my seizures with acquaintances, not knowing whether the person with whom I spoke would begin to see me as less smart, less capable, or less of a human being. Steve had made a different choice. He did not speak about his seizures openly. A nationally recognized intellectual, Steve is one of the most exceptionally kind and bright people I know. He has fought many battles to make a difference in other people's lives; for him, this battle was a solitary one. Steve was worried that on medication he did not think as fast as he had before.

"What makes you believe that?" I asked.

"I don't know. I can't quite remember," he answered, using humor to defend against self-doubts.

"Is there something specific that makes you worry that you are not thinking as fast as before?"

Anxious not to talk soberly about such a serious concern, he continued evasively, "I can't quite put my finger on it that quickly, but give me some time and I'll be able to come up with it."

"How can you say that? You wrote your last book when you were on medication and it's been a blockbuster," argued Rossie, who was surprised by Steve's concerns, despite the closeness of her friendship with him.

Steve did not answer, but I knew the response. "This work was brilliant but the work that was not written would have been even better." Steve smiled when I broke the silence and answered for him, then acknowledged that was how he felt.

"I also can't talk as fast as I could before," he added.

"Steve, that's something different. Not being able to speak fast doesn't mean you're not thinking fast. Not being able to speak fast can be a problem with coordination. One side effect of anticonvulsants is ataxia: you may have poorer coordination. It wouldn't have anything more to do with how fast you think than your typing speed does."

I was feeling comfortable that my intellectual and personal life had not been handicapped by what had happened, though my life had been changed. I was hoping that Steve could feel similarly. I was hoping that he could feel a pride in his remarkable accomplishments that was not tinged with a sense of regret at what might have been.

Though it had been years since his first seizure, Steve still had fundamental gaps in his knowledge of what he could do to help limit his seizures. Steve's persistent questioning revealed his desire to learn, yet no physician treating him had taken the time to explain to him what he needed to know. When Steve had had a seizure recently at night, he did not know that he should tell his doctor about it and get the blood level of his anticonvulsant tested. He did not know that exhaustion could have lowered his seizure threshold; when he learned this, he immediately felt that it was a significant contributor to his last seizure.

If Steve decides one day to proclaim publicly that he lives with epilepsy, he will make a great difference in the lives of those with seizures and the attitudes of many without. In a world where painfully few in public life acknowledge having had seizures, children and adults with epilepsy would have one more model, and those who discriminate would have one more visible opponent. He could begin the process of doing for epilepsy what Betty Ford and Happy Rockefeller did for breast cancer.

Such an acknowledgment would change his life. Some of the changes would undoubtedly be for the better: he would be less isolated and able to learn more about his own seizures from the wide circle of people living with seizures and from people who address the needs of those with epilepsy. But not all the changes would be better for him personally. The price he would pay because of discrimination is difficult to estimate, but discrimination would inevitably happen. One can hear it stated simply in a letter written by a father of a boy with epilepsy, which was sent to members of the Epilepsy Foundation. The father ended his letter: "Daniel is not my son's real name. It's a pseudonym. I'm using [a pseudonym] because of the prejudice that still exists against people with epilepsy. . . . When the time comes, making his condition public will be his decision to make, not mine." He was using a pseudonym even to a friendly audience.

I have been blasted too many times by bigoted comments to recommend disclosure lightly. The price for openness is clearly discrimination in our lifetime. But it has to be done; it is the only hope for equality in the lives of our children.

While I had begun to deal with the daily aspects of living with the risk of seizures, Tim's and my decision about another pregnancy remained. More than a year after the article in the *New England Journal of Medicine* on taking Tegretol during pregnancy had first appeared, the storm the article caused had run its course. Few of the experts with whom Tim and I spoke still believed that Tegretol was dangerous during pregnancy. Limitations in the study's methodology and its overstatement of conclusions had been misleading. Tegretol still had risks, but probably few compared to other anticonvulsants. My neurologist and obstetrician told us it would be relatively safe to go ahead and have another child. Before making a final decision, we made an appointment with a specialist on teratogens, medications that can cause birth defects.

When doctors wonder why patients get multiple opinions, they rarely look at the history of the patient. As is the case in many other families, our uncertainty had been fed by conflicting medical opinions. Two years earlier we had been told that as many as one in five children born to mothers taking Tegretol might be severely affected. Now we were told that the risk of a serious problem was low.

The night before our appointment with the specialist, I dreamt I met our newborn child. The health care providers told me that the bridge of the baby's nose was flat, and that the flattening could be a sign of serious effects from Tegretol exposure. "What about the baby's nails?" I asked, as I looked for hypoplasia, nails that were smaller than normal, another sign of birth defects that could be from the Tegretol. Dreams described more honestly than speech the guilt I still felt about taking medication during pregnancy. During the day, that guilt — irrational, but powerful — was silenced by the perspective of family and friends. I knew I had tried, and physicians had tried with me — through surgery and lowering anticonvulsant doses until seizures struck — to avoid the need to take anticonvulsants during pregnancy.

The following morning Tim and I went to see a specialist at the National Birth Defects Center. She summarized all the research to date, saying the risk of having a child with a problem was low. During the visit, she estimated that one in thirty children exposed to Tegretol in utero would be affected. But she did not put those details in her follow-up letter. She was nervous about the legal risk she would take by putting something so uncertain in writing. She explained that the majority of those affected would be affected only in minor ways, such as by nail hypoplasia. But a few could be seriously affected, with malformed hearts or marked developmental delays.

Tim and I talked about what to do for days. Tim talked about the fact that the fetus would not be exposed to other serious common teratogens, such as cigarette smoke and alcohol, and about the likelihood that the baby would be born healthy. We talked about what the baby's life would be like if something did happen. We thought about how any problem the baby had would also affect Ben's life. We had discussions about what was most important to us, discussions made more difficult by the profound need for honesty with ourselves.

We decided to have another child. We knew that the pregnancy itself could be complicated. For some women who have had seizures, pregnancy increases the chance of further seizures; for other women it decreases the chance or has no effect.

But we thought that becoming pregnant would be easy; it was not. Tim and I were filled with joy when we found out in December that I was pregnant.

JANUARY 1992

Saturday, I slept on and off while Ben watched *Sesame Street*. Tim was on call at the hospital. After weeks of nighttime awakenings, I was exhausted. As I napped, I had nightmares that I could not wake myself up.

Sunday evening, I tried to pour apple juice into Ben's sippy cup and spilled it all over the floor. Later that night the same thing happened with another drink. Monday morning it was the vitamins. After the vitamins fell, I noticed I had left-sided weakness as well as fatigue. Then I realized what was happening. It had never felt right; I had never felt anything slipping. I had lost a split second and all of a sudden things were on the floor. Each time I had the object in my left hand.

At noon on Monday, Martin Luther King Jr.'s birthday, my left hand knocked into my glass, spilling milk on the table. Ben noticed and tried to reassure me. "It's okay, Mommy. We can clean it up. We just need to get some towels."

They were the beginnings of focal seizures brought on by the fatigue and hormonal shifts of pregnancy, stopped before generalizing by the anticonvulsant medication. I had to set limits on what I did. My mother took Ben, and I slept.

JUNE 1992

My parents came to our house at 7:15 in the morning to walk with us to the first celebration, a breakfast for those receiving their Ph.D.s. While a MacArthur Foundation Fellow, I had completed a Ph.D. in public policy. The crimson-and-black doctoral gown billowed over my seven-months-pregnant belly. Ben took my tassel and ran ahead.

At the beginning of the graduation ceremony, President

Rudenstine spoke the usual platitudes. But when he thanked the families for what they had done to help the graduates arrive at where they were, I began to cry. Its truth was far more painfully clear to me than in the past.

That night we returned to Upstairs at the Pudding, where we had had dinner three years earlier on the night of my graduation from medical school. This time I had medication in my pocket and a plate in my head. Yet life was also richer than it had been before. I could not take a bite of the meal without savoring its sweetness.

AUGUST 25, 1992

As my due date passed, my obstetrician grew concerned that the baby might be growing too large before his birth. She worried that giving birth to a large infant might increase my risk of bleeding into my brain again during the delivery. She wanted to induce labor before the baby grew too large, so she ordered an ultrasound to check its size.

After performing the ultrasound in an equipment-filled room, the radiologist left, with a male doctor-in-training trailing him silently. As I began to get dressed in the room left dark during the ultrasound, the technician came in with a picture of our son and the ultrasound report. The baby was small, not large: the biparietal diameter was 1.7 standard deviations below the mean. In other words, the distance from one side of his head to the other was only in the fifth percentile for his age. I stared at the numbers as the darkness of the room reflected what would be our ignorance of their meaning. As I opened the door, the doctor was standing there waiting. Unusual. Normally, patients wait for the doctor out front. He tried awkwardly to play down the worries he anticipated.

"Babies' heads can be small for any number of reasons." Some mean that they will have difficulty for the rest of their

lives; others do not. But if the small head size was due to the
Tegretol, the problem could be significant.

That evening, while Tim went to the local grocery store
with Ben, I read in our pediatric textbooks about "micro-
cephaly," "small for gestational age," and "intrauterine growth
retardation." After Ben's bedtime, I sat down and began to talk
to Tim.

"I'm worried about the baby's size."

"They told us not to worry unless the head size was in the
third percentile or lower," he replied.

"But we both know that the difference between the third
and fifth percentile is an artificial cutoff."

"They never told us anything about Tegretol and small
size."

"I looked it up and —"

"When we talked to the geneticists before, they never
told us anything —"

"It's in the journal articles —"

"Don't interrupt me!"

"I was just trying to explain that there's evidence —"

"You don't like it when I interrupt you."

"You're getting angry at me because something might be
wrong."

"No, I'm angry at you because you're making a big deal
about the test."

We saw the same abyss from opposite sides.

I knew how often children's problems drive a wedge
between parents, how important it was for Tim and me to face
everything together, not taking our pain out on each other.

That night, I kept awakening. By one-thirty in the morning, it was clear I wouldn't sleep. I wanted to talk to Tim. I
thought about tossing and turning to awaken him but instead

brought a book to bed and turned on a bright flashlight purportedly to read.

Tim woke. "Hi. It's a mommy kind of night," he said,
referring to how much difficulty I was having sleeping toward
the end of the pregnancy.

Soon jokes were a temporary tonic for our pain. I fell
back asleep with my head on his chest.

AUGUST 27, 1992

Pediatricians get used to judging infants' sizes with a glance. As
the obstetrician delivered Jeremy and handed him to Tim to
hold for the first time, I blurted out with relief, "He's a big
boy!"

It was just one moment in the long process of having to
take risks to live, but it is one for which I am forever grateful.

WINTER 1992 AND SPRING 1993

On December 1, 1992, I became a faculty member in the
Harvard Medical School Department of Health Care Policy. In
March, I traveled to the Centers for Disease Control in Atlanta
to present research on tuberculosis conducted while a Mac-
Arthur Foundation Fellow. Then Tim and I traveled to an
international symposium in Zurich to present research we had
carried out on the risk of infectious diseases in the blood
supply.

Surgery had not given me my old life back: my life had been
changed forever. But I had given birth to Jeremy, returned to
productive work, and gone back to traveling — not because of
the surgery but because of the unrelenting support of family and
friends, acceptance, adaptation, and persistence driven by profound desire.

A surgical-and-medical cure is not a possibility for most
conditions, and even when it is a possibility, it often fails.

Learning to live with our diseases or chronic conditions is an option we all have. I knew the sound of these words before, but I did not know what they meant; neither the destination nor the road there was familiar. Becoming a doctor had taught me little about the process of living with chronic conditions and diseases despite the fact that that is what most doctors' patients are doing.

As I worked full-time as an assistant professor of health policy and cared for my sons, I wrote. Sometimes I thought about how my colleagues would react to a book full of the stories, not the statistics, of human lives. It was not lost on me that the only sentence the *New England Journal of Medicine* had deleted from my letter was the one that said that I personally had had seizures.

One of my colleagues, an expert in research on patient-doctor relationships, unaware that I was writing this book, showed me a notebook that contained the results of a survey of patients. There were pages and pages of statistics followed by pages of paragraphs patients had written about their experiences.

"You need the statistics, but there are things the stories convey that the statistics can't," he explained.

That is why I kept writing — despite the taboos. Taboos against the lessons of individual human lives, often dismissed as "anecdotal." Taboos against the personal, criticized as not being "objective," as if viewpoints did not affect all our work.

While individual stories do not describe the experience of an entire society, statistics do not fully capture any individual's experience. Surveys cannot tell us anything the authors of the survey do not ask. The questions are limited by time, by multiple-choice answers, and by our prior understanding of the subject. What surveys convey in numbers they lose in important details. What we learn from human stories, lived and told in their full human context, complements what we learn from asking less about more people.

During the day, I worked as a university researcher, looking for answers to questions about our lives in lengthy analyses of short questions asked of thousands nationally. At night, I documented the details of individual lives.

I hoped that writing in the first person would help in the fight to change a medical culture — insulated and steeped in denial — that is nurtured by and reflected in the language doctors use. When physicians say "His squash was really fried," they are purposely placing a distance between themselves and patients. When doctors say "He coded on me," it is as if the patient is injuring the doctor with his heart attack, and that is how it is often perceived when the patient's illness interrupts the sleep of the resident. As we begin to talk more about our own experiences with each other, to use the first person as we speak about what has happened to us, our family members, and our friends, then perhaps more of us will say "My grandfather just coded, and it felt like he was the one who hurt." It would be an important start toward collapsing the distance between patients and physicians. When doctors learn to stop relying solely on the second person in speech, we will spend less time telling patients "You will feel . . ." and more time listening to how patients feel. We will spend less time dictating to patients and more time asking patients what is important to them before giving advice.

MAY 1993

In May, I returned to visit the refugee health projects in southern Mexico. Soon after I arrived, there was a word of an attempted military coup in Guatemala. I spent the early mornings and late evenings huddled with refugees around an unfinished wooden table whose centerpiece was a shortwave radio, listening for news about whether the coup would succeed and what was happening to civilians.

One morning, Armando's wife spoke when we were alone, "This fall it will be three years since Armando disappeared. I'm writing the human rights commission again." She told me of her repeated efforts to get the commission to help find him and her desolation at how little had been done by any officials to determine what had happened to her husband. She knew her efforts had at times endangered her own life.

She told me that the morning of his abduction, Armando awakened feeling sick with the flu. Tamara urged him to stay home and rest, but they needed money, so he insisted on going to the marketplace to try and sell crafts. Tamara waited with their children for him to come home. When he did not come back all day Saturday, she worried he had been in an accident. She went to all the clinics and hospitals asking for him. With tears filling her eyes, she explained that when he was not at any of the clinics, she began to worry that the Mexican police had picked him up. She thought of all the stories she had heard of innocent people being mistaken for drug dealers or being picked up, imprisoned, and tortured.

Tamara's children spent their days asking "Does Daddy have enough to eat? Is Daddy thirsty?" — questions arising from their firsthand experience with bare survival — and saying "When Daddy comes home, I'm going to tell him . . ." But while sleeping, the pain permeating their souls was released in shrieks and screams. They spent the nights crying, unconscious to the fact that their mother spent hours holding them, trying to calm their nightmares of reality.

"The last time anyone had seen him was at noon in the park," Tamara continued. "So we started asking people who worked in between the park and the market if they'd seen him. Then a neighbor heard from a boy who was too frightened to tell any official that at noon, at the truck stop outside the market, he'd seen a man forced into a white Datsun without license plates." Army intelligence and the treasury police had both been reported to use white "death vans" to kidnap and kill civilians charged with no crimes in Guatemala. A branch of the Guatemalan military called G-2 was reported to have secret operations in Tapachula.

Although human rights conditions were far better in Mexico than in Guatemala, they were far from good. People had been reported detained without criminal charges and tortured. In Michoacán State, a town mayor who brought attention to human rights abuses was himself subsequently detained and tortured. The members of commissions that investigated human rights abuses were also not safe. The president of the independent Commission for the Defense of Human Rights in Sinaloa was murdered.

No one except Armando's kidnappers knew why he disappeared. There was no habeas corpus. There was no legal detention. There were never any charges. Many speculated that he was kidnapped because of the health care he provided. At times, as many as a dozen refugees would be at his home receiving care. He could have been kidnapped because he knew the names of the undocumented refugees whom he had helped. Others speculated that he had been politically active eight years ago when he lived in Guatemala.

What Partners in Health knew was a man who had grown up with no formal education but who had managed to learn how to take care of children and adults alike with basic illnesses. Armando shared these skills by teaching other refugees how to provide health care. He was humble and heroic. He continued to care for all those in need despite the great risk to health care workers. He provided that care to refugees for seven years, for as long as he himself had been a refugee. His clothes had patches. He traveled for days at a time to train other health care workers, carrying one small bag with one change of shirt. His family lived with him in a very small home, and his earnings were barely enough to feed and clothe them. That is why he was going to the market to sell crafts that day.

The other health care workers continued to work in the region despite Armando's disappearance, recognizing that their own lives were at risk. Tamara began to learn to work as a health promoter.

On that return visit to the refugee health care program, it was clear that women still faced many barriers to becoming health providers. Helena was one of the few in training. She arrived early at the course for health care workers with all her belongings and those of her son packed in one large purse; she owned two dresses, one to wear while the other hung out to dry. She was the first to arrive yet the last to eat. While she sat caring lovingly and proudly for her nine-month-old, Miguel, the men ate.

We began with the most ordinary words between mothers. "Can I hold Miguel for you while you eat?" I offered as soon as I saw her in the dining room with her by now cold food untouched. As she handed Miguel to me, she asked how old my children were.

Miguel and I were soon cooing at each other and laughing. As Miguel gurgled happily, I talked with Helena about how well Miguel was standing, and speaking, and doing everything babies do.

"What would you do if someone gave you a baby?" she asked suddenly.

"What do you mean?" I asked, stunned.

Hesitating after hearing my answer but unwilling to turn

back if going forward might help her son, she continued, "What would you do if you found a baby left by its mother?"

"I would feel terrible," I explained, choosing my words carefully, realizing that she was talking about herself. "It would be so unspeakably sad for the mother and her child."

Miguel had not left her arms except for the few moments it took her to eat. She adored him. She did not want to give Miguel up for adoption; she feared she would have to out of poverty.

We went outside to talk as she rinsed out a rag diaper full of diarrhea. She explained that she could not find work since Miguel's birth; it was not safe for him in the sweatshops, where she had worked before becoming pregnant. Helena hoped that, after the training, she could earn a living as a health care provider. But even continuing the course with Miguel would be impossible as soon as he was old enough that his bus fare was no longer free. There was no one else to care for him, and the scholarship for the course supplied money for her transportation only.

The economic situation had not improved, but, the training staff explained, many of the large aid organizations were no longer providing help to the refugees. The aid organizations had grown tired of the refugees' problems. The refugees had been in Mexico a decade, many remained desperately poor, and still did not have full legal status. If they returned to Guatemala, they did not know if they could be killed or sent to guarded camps.

Many of the aid organizations were ceasing to serve Mexicans as well. In Chiapas, the lives of indigenous Mexicans bore many parallels to those of the rural Guatemalan *indigenas* who took refuge with them. The aid organizations did not foresee that the disparities in wealth among Mexicans in Chiapas were so corrosive and conditions the poor lived under so inhuman that they would lead to an uprising in January 1994. They saw what they wanted or needed to see.

Helena's question haunted me.

JUNE 1993

Lia and I stood outside having missed our medical school reunion luncheon. We had hardly known each other during medical school. Still, the strength of the bond of having been through the initiation into the fraternity of physicians together made us willing to talk about our lives.

Lia began to talk about why she had almost missed the reunion. "I haven't even been thinking about it these past few weeks. I had meant to go, then forgot we had one. My mom's dying . . ."

"I'm so sorry to hear that. . . ." I meant it.

"We've all been taking turns caring for her . . .

She went on to describe in moving detail how her mother was focusing on getting everything taken care of—from arranging her own funeral to helping her husband accept her death. Then Lia stopped. She began again slowly, softly, struggling, "You know, there's a grieving room in the hospital where I work. We're always trying to move families out of it. I never really understood how important it was. I hope I never forget what this is like. . . . I hope I can keep it with me in my work. I never want to hurry anyone who's grieving again."

Her whole life had been changed—not in the stereotypical way, from callous doctor to sensitive one. Lia had always been sensitive. But like all of us, she had had more to learn about what it means to be a patient and part of a patient's family. Neither had been taught in medical school. She had been trained in a system that was organized around patients, but neither by them nor with their equal participation.

There was only one grieving room where she worked. There was often more demand for the room than space. Instead of changing the space allotment in the hospital, physicians sped patients' families through their losses and life-arresting changes. Physicians have been taught through actions if not words that medicine's first job is curing, even if it means caring is cut short for the many whom doctors are unable to cure.

We said good-bye, and Lia returned to her family. I went back to the office to work until it was time for the evening gathering.

That evening, Ann and I caught up with each other. I was still hungry from having missed lunch and she was four months pregnant, so together we ate our way through the snacks as others drank their way through the beer. Ann had stopped drinking alcohol for the duration of her pregnancy, and I avoided it, knowing it might lower my seizure threshold.

"I had a pregnancy that ended in fetal demise," Ann began. "People sort of expected that after six weeks it'd be fine. That was that. It was over. On to the next thing." She paused. "But I didn't feel that way at all. I felt horrible," she explained, her voice slowing to pronounce each syllable. "It was a real death to me," she said as her speech changed back from the medical jargon of fetal demise to speaking as a mother about death and loss. She lowered her voice as some of our classmates approached.

We had been taught to learn from physicians, not patients. On the way home, I began to wonder about how things might change if instead of confiding quietly to one another doctors spoke aloud about their experiences as patients and as family members in the health care system. And then went further: What if doctors learned from patients as equal partners with physicians from the start?

CHAPTER FOURTEEN

Changing Health Care

The truth, of course, is that many
hospitals have indeed failed to make
patients' needs their primary concern.

—*"News from Harvard Medical, Dental, and
Public Health Schools,"* Focus (1994).

WORKING IN HEALTH CARE POLICY, I rarely mentioned my personal experiences. Knowing that individual experiences were not always representative, and realizing that patients' experiences and knowledge were undervalued by many
physicians, I was hesitant to generalize from individual experience. But my concern about the position in which patients are
placed grew, and my reticence to speak out diminished as more
and more patients and physicians began telling me their stories.

Some of the stories reflected failed relationships at critical
moments in patients' lives. Vivian described telling her obstetrician that she thought her baby was about to be born, that she
could feel the head coming down her vagina. He did not believe
her and so did not do a physical exam. Minutes later, he and
the delivery nurses were unprepared when the baby was born
"precipitously." It was only precipitous to them because the
obstetrician had not listened to Vivian.

Lena had severe lower abdominal pain and a high fever.

Taking a sample of pus with a cotton swab during a pelvic exam would have diagnosed her infection in time. Without the exam she became so ill that a hysterectomy was required in order to save her life.

Many of the stories simply underscored the texture of daily doctor-patient relationships. John, a young physician-in-training, explained that he had scared a patient into believing that she might die if a test was not performed because he was worried that she would not return for the test. He thought it was important for the patient to have the test and believed she wouldn't understand if he just explained why.

Lisa's seizures were getting worse and worse. She was having many every day. She tried to talk with her doctor about how they were affecting her life, and he said, "You have to rise above it." She ceased to talk with doctors about any of the effects seizures had on her health.

Silva had cancer. He was young and had been perfectly healthy a year before. The first physician who cared for him had failed to detect his cancer. When chemotherapy was started, it worked temporarily, but the cancer soon returned. We sat and talked shortly after his relapse. He was one of the patients doctors talk about being pained to see. Silva said simply, "The more training the doctors get, the more they stay away from me and won't talk to me."

While a number of my colleagues, family, and friends had had excellent encounters with physicians, the majority told of times when their symptoms were disbelieved or minimized by physicians; when physicians knew little about what it was like to be a patient with a particular condition or undergoing a specific treatment; when physicians dictated what they should do instead of sharing the decision making; or when the quality of their care and their lives was diminished because of their relationship with the physicians who cared for them.

In medical school, I had read a great deal about what we did well as physicians. As I listened to patients' experiences, I began to read about what we still needed to improve. What I found was that my own experiences and the experiences of those I knew were far from unique. We had in common a desire to know more. In fact, studies show that the overwhelming majority of patients want information about their care (Blanchard, Labrecque, et al. 1988), and there is a direct relationship between how much information patients receive and how satisfied they are (Hall, Roter, and Katz 1988). Yet physicians seriously underestimate the amount of information patients want (Faden, Lewis, et al. 1981; Faden, Becker, et al. 1981). Those patients who want information about their medical care continue to experience the greatest disparities between what they would hope for in their care and what care they receive (Cleary, Edgman-Levitan, et al. 1992). Even the fact that patients change doctors when their doctors are unwilling to spend time talking with them (Kasteller, Kane, et al. 1976) has not changed the profession.

If doctor-patient relations are problematic for patients who are white middle-class men, they are far more so for those patients who are poor, for people of color, and for women. Studies show how common disparities in treatment are: whites receive more care than people of color (Goldberg, Hartz, et al. 1992; Braveman, Oliva, et al. 1989; Todd, Samaroo, et al. 1993; Ayanian, Udvarhelyi, et al. 1993); men get more care than women (Ayanian and Epstein 1991; Steingart, Packer, et al. 1991); women are given less information and fewer choices than men (Stevens 1992). Studies have also found that low-income patients receive poorer-quality care (Newacheck 1989). This occurs even when they have health insurance. Jessy, Caitlin, and I were all treated as if we were uncooperative or lying when we were seen for seizures in an emergency room. But when physicians in the emergency room found out that my husband and I were both physicians, they realized I was just confused from the seizure, and my care improved. Caitlin, a black woman with a developmental disability who came in alone, was sent home without care only to have another seizure.

Even when patients receive care, discrimination affects doctor-patient communication. A national survey of patients found communication problems were most frequent between doctors and low-income patients, those belonging to a minority, and those in poorest health (Cleary, Edgman-Levitan, et al. 1991). One Hispanic colleague went to an emergency room complaining of severe right lower quadrant pain, saying he had appendicitis. He was labeled a "hysterical Hispanic" until his appendix ruptured twenty-four hours later. Discriminatory stereotypes are passed down from physicians to medical students in anecdotes and passed off as humor. Furthermore, physicians are less likely to practice "partnership-building" with or provide information to patients who are poor or have less advanced education (Street 1992; Brody 1980).

"Informed consent" is often little more than uninformed acquiescence. Dr. Barrows spent time discussing the surgery with me in detail but during my hospitalizations consent for medical care was covered by a global statement: "Permission is given to the University Hospitals, Inc., and its physicians, employees, agents and servants for the performance of any diagnostic examination, treatment, biopsy, transfusion and/or surgical procedure, and for the administration of any anesthetic that may be deemed advisable in the course of this hospital admission."

The limited discussions physicians had with me about the medications they prescribed paralleled what I witnessed in medical school and internship but were in sharp contrast to the research on what patients would like. Ninety-eight percent of patients want to know the side effects of their treatment, and

99 percent want to know "what the treatment will accomplish." More than 95 percent want to know "exactly what the treatment will do inside my body" and almost as many want to know "what the day-to-day (or week-to-week) progress is" (Cassileth, Zupkis, et al. 1980). Far more patients than doctors believe that patients should choose among treatment options (Faden, Becker, et al. 1981). Even among those patients who do not want to make final decisions about their treatment options, the overwhelming majority want to learn in detail about their health problems and possible treatments, including their benefits and side effects (Kessler 1991).

When I met Jerid in the Children's Hospital emergency room, he hungered for information about what was happening to him and his broken arm. Children, like Jerid, are not told what is happening; their parents are often also left in the dark (Able-Boone, Dokecki, and Smith 1989). Among mothers who take their sick child to the pediatrician, 45 percent leave not knowing what treatment their child should receive, and 30 percent leave not knowing when their child should return to be checked by the doctor (Decastro 1972). While 52 percent of parents have stated that they need to know more about their child's diagnosis, and 54 percent about their child's treatment, only 8 percent of physicians think parents need more information about children's diagnoses, and only 3 percent of physicians think that parents need more information about children's treatments (Liptak and Revell 1989). Wanting to be told more is not unique to relatives of patients in the United States. While relatives of patients in intensive care units in Great Britain rate it as very important to "have explanations given in understandable terms" and to "have . . . questions answered honestly," only 37 percent and 42 percent respectively, expect that their doctors will do so (McIvor and Thompson 1988).

Some doctors argue that sharing information about side

effects and sharing decisions will make patients more likely to experience side effects, not "comply" with treatment, or just be more "anxious." Research demonstrates the opposite (Quaid 1990; Todd 1989; Baird-Lambert and Buchanan 1985). Patients are most likely to follow recommendations from physicians who inform them about their illnesses and treatment, demonstrate that they respect patients and understand their concerns, and involve them in developing a plan for treatment (Stoeckle 1993; Todd 1989; Jones 1983; Baird-Lambert and Buchanan 1985).

Furthermore, patients who are allowed to take an active role in their own care experience more satisfaction with their medical care (Brody, Miller, et al. 1989; Lewis, Pantell, and Sharp 1991; Kaplan 1993). Spending even a brief period of time encouraging patients to become more involved in making decisions about their own care and teaching patients to understand their medical records and their diseases has been shown to ameliorate patients' health (Greenfield, Kaplan, and Ware 1985). Improvements in health that result from increased patient participation can be measured in laboratory tests as well as in decreased symptoms (Greenfield, Kaplan, et al. 1988; Kaplan, Greenfield, and Ware 1989).

Those opposed to giving patients an equal voice in their care have argued that when given information about a range of options for care, patients will always choose the most expensive option. That fear has not been borne out by research. When given information about surgical and medical treatments by fellow patients who have experienced both treatments, more patients with an enlarged prostate selected the less expensive medical management — even though the patients were fully insured and would not pay the difference in cost (Kasper, Mulley, and Wennberg 1992).

Involving patients in their own care has been shown to lead

to a variety of direct cost savings. Patients who received more information about their care have been found to require less pain medication, recover more rapidly, and spend fewer days in the hospital (Kaplan and Ware 1989). Both high blood pressure and high blood sugar — conditions that can lead to ill health and the need for expensive care — have been shown to be significantly better controlled after increasing the role patients play in their own medical care (Greenfield, Kaplan, et al. 1988). In addition, enlarging the role patients play in their own care has been shown to lead to lower indirect costs, such as the number of work days lost (Kaplan, Greenfield, and Ware 1989).

In order to change doctor-patient relationships, we will need to change medical education. Medical students, residents, and attendings alike often see little of patients' lives and may not understand what they do see. Postoperative recovery is just one example. Patients recovering do not go directly from lying down to walking, yet the snapshots physicians currently see belie this fact. Physicians see patients first in the hospital at their sickest, in critical care; the next time doctors see patients, they are often walking and talking, at follow-up checkups commonly six weeks or two months after surgery. Although physicians know little about the majority of patients' recovery, medical students and new physicians commonly learn about patients' experiences from other physicians rather than from patients. The message physicians give each other about patients' experience is often inaccurate at the beginning and, as in a game of "telephone tag," the message gets more distorted each time it is passed along. The personal experiences of individual doctors who happen to become patients will not transform medical education. The majority of young and middle-aged physicians will not have a serious illness until they have taught and practiced medicine for years; nor would I ever wish such an experience on them.

Not only do students miss learning about patients' lives, but students are taught by example to treat patients as less than equals. They are taught that patients have fewer rights than physicians and medical students. One student was upset after a teacher had him examine an unconscious patient. He later spoke to his instructor about his apprehension that the patient, comatose, could not be given a choice about being "used as a teaching case." The instructor brushed off his concerns, saying, "This is a teaching hospital, so patients don't have any choice." In fact, by law they do.

Students are taught they should interview and examine patients regardless of the patient's wishes. Andy was frustrated with a ward patient in pain who would not talk with him. He wanted to know how to get patients like this woman to "let me interview them." I remember so often hearing that question as a medical student. The possibility of respecting a sick patient's desire not to be interviewed by students was rarely raised. Equally rare was Tim's commonsense answer: "Help with her pain first."

Students are taught to involve patients in treatment decisions only enough to obtain formal consent, not to provide real choices. Third-year medical students — still willing to describe what they see honestly — detail this process and how it fails patients. Michael, weeks into his first rotation in surgery, said what we all knew was true: "When the surgeons send you in to get informed consent, they're just sending you in to get a signature. They don't want you to talk to the patient about what's really involved in the surgery or what all the different complications might be because they don't want you to mess up the schedule. If you get the patient all concerned, then a surgeon will have to go in and have a long talk with the patient about what's going to happen, and the patient might even change his mind."

When patients are unhappy with their role, many doctors

teach students that the fault lies with the patient. One article typifies this attitude. In discussing the "angry, demanding, complaining" patient, the authors say: "The behavior of these patients arises from an unreasonable and exaggerated fear that they will not get what they need." The authors do not even raise the possibility that perhaps the patient had unhappy experiences in the health care system, or has reasonable concerns and real fears. The article advises that "the physician can retain control of the situation by letting the patient know what will and will not be tolerated" (Schwenk and Romano 1992).

The problems with these attitudes and practices are clear to medical students at the beginning of their clinical training. Medical students and interns stand at the precipice, still identifying closely with the patients. But in their position as apprentices, they seek the approval necessary to succeed and learn to copy the behavior of more senior physicians. One study showed that early in their training interns interrupted patients almost half the time before the patients finished the opening description of their concerns. As time went on, interns "learned" to interrupt more, not less (Meuleman and Harward 1992).

In medical training, as medical students and residents imitate those only slightly more senior, they are taught to see patients as "others." The change can be insidious. A colleague, hospitalized during her last year of medical school, described the shock of going from identifying primarily with doctors to identifying with patients again. A physician who acquired AIDS as a resident while caring for patients wrote poignantly of this experience: "It hit me violently that I had lost sight of my patients as human beings and had begun to see them as a different species: the patient species. I had begun to detach myself from the most important aspect of medicine" (Aoun 1992). Another physician described this loss of empathy for patients during medical training: "As I know them, college students start out with much empathy and genuine love — a real desire to help other people. In medical school, however, they learn to mask their feelings, or worse, to deny them. They learn detachment . . . to focus not on patients, but on diseases" (Spiro 1992).

When doctor-patient relationships are discussed in medical education, it is often far from hospital wards and outpatient clinics. At Harvard, third-year medical students attend a two-hour-a-week course on doctor-patient relationships and work more than eighty hours a week as apprentices on the hospital wards. Throughout the year, students speak about the disparity between the respect for and equality of patients discussed in class and what they see happen in the hospital. One year, this disparity was reflected in the final class project, a film in which third-year students sought to examine student roles in the hospital. The students interviewed other third-year students, residents, and attendings on the wards. Although the course was about patient-doctor relations, they had failed even to include patients' points of view.

We desperately need to change physician training in all settings. Classroom-based courses designed to improve doctor-patient relationships cannot succeed without changing education on the wards and in the clinics. It is time to expand the ways in which patients teach doctors. Doctors have long learned about clinical manifestations of disease from patients. Medical students and doctors need to learn more on the wards, in clinics, and in the community about the experience of illness and health care from patients.

Not only does medical education shape doctor-patient relationships, but so too does research, by affecting what we know and what patient care and health policies are recommended. At present the vast majority of research is designed and presented without the participation of the patients it affects. The people most directly affected by the research are absent not only physically, but their perspective is lacking as well. There are exceptions: one is the field of AIDS, where activist patients, through their protests, have forced physicians to open the doors of research meetings. The presence of people living with AIDS at meetings discussing research leaves an indelible stamp, a constant reminder of how the proposed research affects the lives of individuals. Their presence affects the subjects that are proposed for study, the design of research proposals, interpretations, and policy recommendations based on the results.

The contrast with a meeting on tuberculosis is stark. A group of researchers and policymakers presented a proposal to require every single person who is diagnosed with tuberculosis to have a health care professional present for each pill they take in treatment. They argued that the imposition on infected individuals was trivial and the public health gains great. I sat in the audience and thought about how "directly observed therapy" would take place. Would a health care worker go to the home of the patient twice a week for nine months? That might create one of the lesser burdens but it would be costly to the state and was unlikely to be funded. Would the person with tuberculosis be required to go to the doctor's office or clinic daily? I imagined a common scenario: a mother with two children, with no one to share their care, lives a long distance by public transportation from the clinic; it takes her and her children hours to make each round-trip to the clinic so someone can watch her take a pill she can take on her own at home. I raised my hand to ask for a discussion of the specifics, but I was not called on. I thought about standing up in the meeting and asking how many people in the audience had ever had tuberculosis and whether they could imagine how the proposals would have affected their lives. Would they still feel the public health benefit outweighed the human costs?

After the session, I went to find one of the major proponents of the proposal and asked her what way of implementing directly observed therapy was advocated. "Oh, any way would be fine," she responded. I raised my concern that some means, likely to be adopted because they were cheapest for the state, would not be a "trivial imposition" on patients. The speaker said her group had not thought that the details made a difference. Committed and well meaning, she sincerely seemed to regret the omission. Had a number of individuals with tuberculosis been present, representing a range of personal experiences and perspectives, I doubt the proposers would have stood so strongly behind recommendations so vague that they could have such vastly different impacts on the lives of families.

Research would change — in content as well as in recommendations — if it were based on patients' values and needs. Intended and unintended effects of treatments would be studied in greater detail. There are already simple, reliable measures of patients' experiences after surgery (Cleary, Greenfield, and McNeil 1991). These measures have been used for medical as well as surgical patients (Jette, Davies, et al. 1986). They could be used to give doctors a better understanding of how treatments (their intended and unintended outcomes) affect patients' abilities to care for themselves daily, to eat, dress, bathe, walk, use public transportation, drive, work, spend time with other people, and feel.

If research were based on patients' values and needs, the subjects studied would be expanded. For example, patients repeatedly raise concerns about the side effects of long-term use of medications. We know next to nothing about the long-term consequences of either medical or surgical treatments, yet research still focuses on the short-term benefits and side effects of treatments. Research funding and institutions are not structured to facilitate long-term research.

If doctors and patients were equal partners, research questions would be framed differently. Physicians developing in vitro fertilization studied how many patients who had made it to the stage of embryo transplants went on to have positive pregnancy tests. While those numbers are important, they do not address the question most patients have: If we try in vitro fertilization, what are our chances of giving birth to a baby? Some patients who try in vitro fertilization do not make it to the stage of an embryo transplant, and not everyone who has a positive pregnancy test is able to carry the fetus to term and give birth to a live baby.

Finally, the economics of health care dramatically affect doctor-patient relationships. While there are significant differences in the care patients receive in different settings (Schlesinger, Cleary, and Blumenthal 1989; Marcus and Stone 1984; Hickson, Altemeier, and Perrin 1987), increasingly both physicians practicing in health maintenance organizations and those in fee-for-service settings are placed under financial pressure to limit services to patients, including services they believe are medically necessary. In some hospitals, fee-for-service physicians may lose admitting privileges, on which their practice depends, if too many of their patients are admitted without the ability to pay or without insurance, or stay past the time their insurance covers (Morreim 1988). Physicians working in some health maintenance organizations are penalized if they recommend more visits to specialists and diagnostic tests for patients than their colleagues do. In one extreme case, a managed care organization pays each primary care doctor a fixed fee for all the care any given patient requires. If the patient needs a specialist to consult or an endoscopy to be performed, and the doctor recommends one, the primary care doctor pays for the test or consultation out of his own pocket. If he does not recommend one, he pays nothing.

When doctors are asked to ration care, some patients may never learn the unabridged truth about the risks and benefits of treatment options. In this environment, patients need advocates to provide unbiased information about their options (Moore 1989). Dr. Norman Selverstone, a primary care physician with more than forty years' experience, notes, "If people are being sued for a small amount of money, they make sure they have a lawyer who is on their side who does everything possible within the confines of the law to help them. But if their life is on the line, they may have no advocate. The doctor may be the insurer's advocate, with his eyes on the cost."

The time needed to care for patients is not available in many health care settings. A physician, invited to speak at a Harvard Medical School symposium on doctor-patient relationships after she had lived with cancer, spoke of being unable to return to the health maintenance organization where she had previously worked. Her inability stemmed not from any change in her health, but from a change in her understanding of what it meant to be a patient. She spoke of the importance of spending time with patients, of getting to know them in order to provide good care, and about how that was impossible in the place she had previously worked. A large study found that in health maintenance organizations, waiting time for scheduling an appointment was longer than in the offices of solo practitioners. In addition, waits in the office were protracted, less time was spent with the doctor, and less good explanations were provided of the care that was being given (Rubin, Gandek, et al. 1993).

But the problems are not limited to health maintenance organizations. Many fee-for-service physicians are paid over ten times more an hour for performing simple surgery on anesthetized patients than other doctors are for examining and talking to conscious patients about their symptoms and their diagnostic and therapeutic choices. This has meant that far fewer doctors have gone into primary care, and that those who are in primary care cannot spend enough time with their patients.

Overall, nearly half of all outpatient visits provided by any physician last less than ten minutes, and the average visit lasts just twelve minutes (Stoeckle 1987; Todd 1989). Pediatricians — among the lowest paid of all physicians — commonly spend less than ten minutes with a child and family. In less than ten minutes, the pediatrician needs to assess and discuss the child's physical health, mental health, and development as well as parenting issues, and perform screening tests and give vaccinations.

When doctors are asked their views privately, many say they do not have the time to incorporate patients in decision making. A study of residents found that the average amount of time spent with patients being admitted to the hospital was only seventeen to thirty-one minutes (Lurie, Rank, et al. 1989).

In many areas of medicine, the time spent talking to patients is often inversely proportional to one's seniority. The fact that the most junior medical student often spends the most time with the patient is captured in the advice passed on to students and interns: "Read the medical student's history, the intern's physical exam, the resident's assessment, and the attending's plan." The irony lies not only in the fact that physicians and doctors-in-training are instructed to read the most junior person's note to learn what the patient said, but also in the fact that they are instructed to learn the diagnostic and treatment plans from the people who may spend the least time with the patient.

Doctors' appointments need to be set up to last more than an average of twelve minutes so that physicians can learn that they can afford to listen and that their patients cannot afford for them not to listen. When doctors spend more time with patients, not only can they provide better care, but they can save the cost of unnecessary tests and interventions, which often inadequately and expensively replace communication. They can also save the costs of avoidable misdiagnosis, mistreatment, and patient misunderstanding that lie in the wake of dispatch.

To participate as an equal partner in his or her own care, every person needs to be able to get medical care. Currently, forty million Americans have no health insurance. They see doctors only when they are sickest and have the financial means. Too many hospitals have transferred patients because of their inability to pay, endangering every aspect of the patient's care (Miles 1992).

Continuity is critical to patients' ability to play an active role. Any health care system that is set up in such a way that many people have to change their doctors when they change jobs, retire, or become unemployed is organized to fail patients.

Not only should patients be included in decisions about their own health care, but decisions about the series of changes that will take place in the financing and organization of health care nationwide over the coming decade should include patients. Doctors are ignorant of too many aspects of illness and of patients' lives to work alone.

They need equal partners.

References

Able-Boone, H., P. R. Dokecki, and M. S. Smith. 1989. Parent and Health Care Provider Communication and Decision Making in the Intensive Care Nursery. *Children's Health Care* 18:133–141.

Aoun, H. 1992. From the Eye of the Storm, with the Eyes of a Physician. *Annals of Internal Medicine* 116 (4 [Feb. 15]):335–338.

Ayanian, J. Z. 1993. Heart Disease in Black and White. *New England Journal of Medicine* 329:656–658.

Ayanian, J. Z., and A. M. Epstein. 1991. Differences in the Use of Procedures Between Men and Women Hospitalized for Coronary Heart Disease. *New England Journal of Medicine* 325:222–225.

Ayanian, J. Z., I. S. Udvarhelyi, C. A. Gatsonis, C. L. Pashos, and A. M. Epstein. 1993. Racial Differences in the Use of Revascularization Procedures After Coronary Angiography. *Journal of the American Medical Association* 269:2642–2646.

Baird-Lambert, J., and N. Buchanan. 1985. Compliance with Medication Regimens in Children: Can It Be Improved? *The Medical Journal of Australia* 142:201–203.

Benson, H. A., Jr., and S. A. Dabbert. 1980. A Pilot Project to Forestall Chronic Unemployment Among Young People with Epilepsy. In Wada, J. A., and J. K. Penry, eds. *Advances in Epileptology: The Tenth Epilepsy International Symposium*. New York: Raven Press.

Blanchard, C. G., M. S. Labrecque, J. C. Ruckdeschel, and E. B. Blanchard. 1988. Information and Decision-Making Preferences of Hospitalized Adult Cancer Patients. *Social Science and Medicine* 27:1139–1145.

Braveman, P., F. Oliva, M. G. Miller, R. Reiter, and S. Egerter. 1989. Adverse Outcomes and Lack of Health Insurance Among Newborns in an Eight-County Area of California, 1982–1986. *New England Journal of Medicine* 321:508–513.

Brody, D. S. 1980. The Patient's Role in Clinical Decision Making. *Annals of Internal Medicine* 93:718–722.

Brody, D. S., S. M. Miller, C. E. Lerman, D. G. Smith, and G. C. Caputo. 1989. Patient Perception of Involvement in Medical Care. *Journal of General Internal Medicine* 4:506–511.

Calkins, D. R., L. V. Rubenstein, P. D. Cleary, A. R. Davies, A. M. Jette, A. Fink, J. Kosecoff, R. T. Young, R. H. Brook, and T. L. Delbanco. 1991. Failure of Physicians to Recognize Functional Disability in Ambulatory Patients. *Annals of Internal Medicine* 114:451–453.

Cassileth, B. R., R. V. Zupkis, K. Sutton-Smith, and V. March. 1980. Information and Participation Preferences Among Cancer Patients. *Annals of Internal Medicine* 92:832–836.

Cleary, P. D., S. Edgman-Levitan, M. Roberts, T. W. Moloney, W. McMullen, J. D. Walker, and T. L. Delbanco. Patients Evaluate Their Hospital Care: A National Survey. *Health Affairs* 9:254–267.

Cleary, P. D., S. Edgman-Levitan, W. McMullen, and T. L. Delbanco. 1992. The Relationship Between Reported Problems and Patient Summary Evaluations of Hospital Care. *Quality Review Bulletin* 18:53–59.

Cleary, P. D., S. Greenfield, and B. J. McNeil. 1991. Assessing Quality of Life After Surgery. *Controlled Clinical Trials* 12:189S–203S.

The Commonwealth Fund Survey of Women's Health: Key Tables. 1993. Louis Harris and Associates, Inc.

Decastro, F. J. 1972. Exploring the Effectiveness of Care in a Primary Care Clinic. *Clinical Pediatrics* 11:86–87.

Delbanco, T. L. 1992. Enriching the Doctor-Patient Relationship by Inviting the Patient's Perspective. *Annals of Internal Medicine* 116:414–418.

Dougherty, C. J. 1992. Ethical Values at Stake in Health Care Reform. *Journal of the American Medical Association* 268:2409–2412.

Faden, R. R., C. Becker, C. Lewis, J. Freeman, and A. I. Faden. 1981. Disclosure of Information to Patients in Medical Care. *Medical Care* 19:718–733.

Faden, R. R., C. Lewis, C. Becker, A. I. Faden, and J. Freeman. 1981. Disclosure Standards and Informed Consent. *Journal of Health Politics, Policy and Law* 6:255–284.

Goldberg, K. C., A. J. Hartz, S. J. Jacobsen, H. Krakauer, and A. A. Rimm. 1992. Racial and Community Factors Influencing Coronary Artery Bypass Graft Surgery Rates for All 1986 Medicare Patients. *Journal of the American Medical Association* 267:1473–1477.

Greenfield, S., S. Kaplan, and J. E. Ware. 1985. Expanding Patient Involvement in Care: Effects on Patient Outcomes. *Annals of Internal Medicine* 102:520–528.

Greenfield, S., S. Kaplan, J. E. Ware, E. M. Yano, and H. J. Frank. 1988. Patients' Participation in Medical Care: Effects on Blood Sugar Control and Quality of Life in Diabetes. *Journal of General Internal Medicine* 3:448–457.

Hacib, A. 1992. From the Eye of the Storm, with the Eyes of a Physician. *Annals of Internal Medicine* 116:335–338.

Hall, J., D. L. Roter, and N. R. Katz. 1988. Meta-Analysis of Correlates of Provider Behavior in Medical Encounters. *Medical Care* 26:657–672.

Hickson, G. B., W. A. Altemeier, and J. M. Perrin. 1987. Physician Reimbursement by Salary or Fee-for-Service: Effect on Physician Practice Behavior in a Randomized Prospective Study. *Pediatrics* 80(3):344–350.

Jette, A. M., A. R. Davies, P. D. Cleary, D. R. Calkins, L. V. Rubenstein, A. Fink, J. Koseoff, R. T. Young, R. H. Brook, and T. L. Delbanco. 1986. The Functional Status Questionnaire: Reliability and Validity When Used in Primary Care. *Journal of General Internal Medicine* 1:143–149.

Jones, J. G. 1983. Compliance with Pediatric Therapy: A Selective Review and Recommendations. *Clinical Pediatrics* 22:262–265.

Kaplan, S. 1992. The Future of Patient Input into Medical Decision Making. *Quality Review Bulletin* 18:182.

Kaplan, S. 1993. Enlarging Patient Responsibility. *Forum* 14(3 [July]): 9–11.

Kaplan, S. H., S. Greenfield, and J. E. Ware. 1989. Assessing the Effects of Physician-Patient Interactions on the Outcomes of Chronic Disease. *Medical Care* 3(supplement):S110–S127.

Kaplan, S. H., and J. E. Ware. 1989. The Patient's Role in Health Care and Quality Assessment. In *Providing Quality Care,* 27–68. Philadelphia: American College of Physicians.

Kasper, J. F., A. G. Mulley, and J. E. Wennberg. 1992. Developing Shared Decision-Making Programs to Improve the Quality of Health Care. *Quality Review Bulletin* 18:183–190.

256 References

Kasteler, J., R. L. Kane, D. M. Olsen, and C. Thetford. 1976. Issues Underlying Prevalence of "Doctor-Shopping" Behavior. *Journal of Health and Social Behavior* 17:328–339.

Kessler, D. A. 1991. Communicating with Patients About Their Medications. *New England Journal of Medicine* 325:1650–1652.

Lewis, C. C., R. H. Pantell, and L. Sharp. 1991. Increasing Patient Knowledge, Satisfaction, and Involvement: Randomized Trial of a Communication Intervention. *Pediatrics* 88:351–358.

Liptak, G. S., and G. M. Revell. 1989. Community Physician's Role in Case Management of Children with Chronic Illnesses. *Pediatrics.* 84:465–471.

Lurie, N., B. Rank, C. Parenti, T. Woolley, and W. Snoke. 1989. How Do House Officers Spend Their Nights? A Time Study of Internal Medicine House Staff on Call. *New England Journal of Medicine* 320:1673–1677.

McIvor, D., and F. J. Thompson. 1988. The Self-Perceived Needs of Family Members with a Relative in the Intensive Care Unit (ICU). *Intensive Care Nursing* 4:139–145.

Marcus, A. C., and J. P. Stone. 1984. Mode of Payment and Identification with a Regular Doctor: A Prospective Look at Reported Use of Services. *Medical Care* 22:647–657.

Martin, K. I. 1979. Preferences of Patients and the Fallacy of the Five-Year Survival: Letter to the Editor. *New England Journal of Medicine* 300:927–928.

Meuleman, J. R., and M. P. Harward. 1992. Assessing Medical Interview Performance: Effect of Interns' Gender and Month of Training. *Archives of Internal Medicine* 152:1677–1680.

Miles, S. H. 1992. What Are We Teaching About Indigent Patients? *Journal of the American Medical Association* 268:2561–2562.

Moore, C. 1989. Need for a Patient Advocate. *Journal of the American Medical Association* 262:259–260.

Morreim, E. H. 1988. Cost Containment: Challenging Fidelity and Justice. *Hastings Center Report* 18:20–25.

Newacheck, P. W. 1989. Improving Access to Health Services for Adolescents from Economically Disadvantaged Families. *Pediatrics* 84:1056–1063.

Purrington, W. A. 1911. Reporting Venereal Diseases to the Health Department: From a Legal Standpoint. *Social Diseases* 2(2):29.

Quaid, K. A., R. R. Faden, E. P. Vining, and J. M. Freeman. 1990.

Informed Consent for a Prescription Drug: Impact of Disclosed Information on Patient Understanding and Medical Outcomes. *Patient Education and Counseling* 15:249–259.

Register, C. 1987. *Living with Chronic Illness: Days of Patience and Passion.* New York: Bantam Books.

Rubin, H. R., B. Gandek, W. H. Rogers, M. Kosinski, C. A. McHorney, and J. E. Ware. 1993. Patients' Ratings of Outpatient Visits in Different Practice Settings: Results from the Medical Outcomes Study. *Journal of the American Medical Association* 270:835–840.

Schlesinger, M., P. D. Cleary, and D. Blumenthal. 1989. The Ownership of Health Facilities and Clinical Decisionmaking. *Medical Care* 27:244–257.

Schwenk, T. L., and S. E. Romano. 1992. Managing the Difficult Physician-Patient Relationship. *American Family Physician* 46:1503–1509.

Spiro, H. 1992. What Is Empathy and Can It Be Taught? *Annals of Internal Medicine* 116(10 [May 15]):843–846.

Starr, P. 1982. *The Social Transformation of American Medicine.* New York: Basic Books.

Steingart, R. M., M. Packer, P. Hamm, M. E. Coglianese, B. Gersh, E. M. Geltman, J. Sollano, S. Katz, L. Moye, L. L. Basta, et al. 1991. Sex Differences in the Management of Coronary Artery Disease. *New England Journal of Medicine* 325:226–230.

Stevens, C. 1992. When Doctors Don't Take Them Seriously or Prescribe Drugs Tested Only on Men, Women Are Still Second-Class Patients. *The Washingtonian* 27(6 [June]):75–98.

Stoeckle, J. D. 1993. Improving Communication with Patients. *Forum* 14(3 [July]):7–8.

Street, R. L. 1992. Communicative Styles and Adaptation in Physician-Parent Consultations. *Social Science and Medicine* 34:1155–1163.

Tan, M. W. 1993. Is Good Communication a Vaccination Against Claims? *Forum* 14(3[July]):2.

Todd, K. H., N. Samaroo, and J. R. Hoffman. 1993. Ethnicity as a Risk Factor for Inadequate Emergency Department Analgesia. *Journal of the American Medical Association* 269:1537–1539.

Walsh, James J. 1911. Reporting Venereal Diseases to the Health Department: From a Legal Standpoint. *Social Diseases* 2(2):29.

Wortsman, J. 1979. Preferences of Patients and the Fallacy of the Five-Year Survival: Letter to the Editor. *New England Journal of Medicine* 300:928.